Redford Township District Library
25320 West Six Mile Road
Redford, MI 48240

www.redford.lib.mi.us

Hours:

Mon–Thur 10–8:30
Fri–Sat 10–5
Sunday (School Year) 12–5

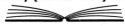

My Feet Are Killing Me!

Dr. Levine's Complete Foot Care Program

Suzanne M. Levine, D.P.M.

McGraw-Hill Book Company

New York   St. Louis   San Francisco   Toronto
Hamburg   Mexico

Whether or not they are beneficial to your feet, no program of strenuous exercises should be undertaken without first consulting the physician who looks after your general health.

2 3 4 5 6 7 8 9 DOC DOC 8 7

ISBN 0-07-037458-9

Library of Congress Cataloging-in-Publication Data

Levine, Suzanne M.
  My feet are killing me!

  1. Foot—Care and hygiene.   2. Foot—Diseases—
Popular works.   I. Title.
RD563.L39   1987   617'.585052   86-19985
ISBN 0-07-037458-9

Exercises for back care reprinted by permission of Riker Laboratories, Inc.

Chart I from *The Foot Book: Healing the Body through Foot Reflexology*, by Devaki Berkson (Funk & Wagnalls) Copyright © 1977 by Devaki Berkson. Reprinted by permission of Harper & Row, Publishers, Inc.

Drawings of footwear through the ages courtesy of The Footwear Council.

Illustrations by Laura Hartman
Book design by Sharen DuGoff Egana
Editing Supervisor: Margery Luhrs

Contents

In Appreciation

Several individuals helped tremendously in putting this foot-pampering book together. I would like to thank Dr. Michael J. Colin for his insights on arthritis. Dr. Colin is a board-certified rheumatologist and internist in private practice in New York City. He holds a teaching appointment at the Mount Sinai School of Medicine in New York and is an attending physician at the Hospital for Joint Diseases—Orthopedic Institute and Beth Israel Medical Center in New York. He is co-chief of the Arthritis Clinic at the Hospital for joint Diseases Orthopedic Institute. He completed his rheumatology training at New York University Medical Center.

I would also like to thank Dr. Harry Schanzer for his section on how blood flow affects the feet. Dr. Schanzer is a board-certified surgeon specializing in vascular diseases and is in private practice in New York. He is an associate professor of surgery at Mount Sinai School of Medicine and director of their Vascular Laboratory.

Thanks are also due to the typists and researchers: Carolyn Krinsley, Carolyn Kitch, Elizabeth Marshall, Mary Beth D'Amico, Jane Pratt, Mary Stein, and Andrew Postman. In addition, I couldn't have completed this manuscript without Dr. Linda Bubbers, Dr. Darlene Courniotis, Dr. Stephen Donis, James Pascarella, Maryann Tinsley, Emma Sanfillippo, Jeannette Alicea, and the rest of my hard-working staff.

I'd also like to thank my husband, Bart, my daughters, Marisa and Heather, and my parents, Maurice and Miriam Marin.

Introduction

Fact: 87 percent of all Americans suffer from foot ailments, and the vast majority accept their pain as a fact of life. "My feet are killing me" is an expression heard in all seasons from all sorts of people.

Fact: In 1985 alone, $200 million was spent on a myriad of over-the-counter remedies purported to relieve or cure foot aches and pains. Athlete's foot powders and ointments accounted for $47 million, and more than $86 million was spent on salves and pads.

Fact: The average person who buys new shoes tries to stretch them to fit unaverage feet. Needless to say, this never works. My patients have closets full of nearly new shoes that all "kill" their feet.

Fact: There are no books on the market now to advise you on keeping your feet healthy no matter what shoes you prefer, to give you advice on treating everyday aches, or to evaluate the incredible array of foot-pampering products available to you.

PART ONE

Levine's Law:
It's Not Normal for Feet to Hurt!

Chapter 1
Walking Proof of
My Own Pampering Programs

Feet have been a focal point of my life for as long as I can remember. I have made peace with these troublesome parts of my body, but isn't it remarkable that I can't remember when my feet weren't on my mind, for better or for worse? My own experience is the reason I wrote this book for you.

My mother tells me that by the age of two, I was a regular patient at the Hospital for the Ruptured and Disabled in New York City (now part of the Hospital for Special Surgery). At this dire-sounding place I was fitted with my first pair of orthopedic shoes. They were supposed to correct my very bowed baby legs, which were causing me problems in learning to walk. Those cumbersome shoes only added to my difficulties. Looking back, both my mother and I blame my chubby, inactive early childhood on a congenital foot abnormality.

By the time I turned five, Suzanne's special shoes with the prescription arches, the orthopedic "cookies," with their complete lack of little-girl appeal were a regular topic of family conversation. How I hated them. My parents insisted that my very flat, very wide feet and developing bunion needed all the podiatric assistance they could get. It was for my own good.

But I didn't care. I wanted sneakers and I wanted black patent "Mary Janes." I wanted the kinds of shoes other girls my age were wearing. Besides, those big, brown oxfords made it almost impossible for me to run or jump (try picking one up). Given my feelings and the expense of the shoes, the regular shoe-shopping trips were an ordeal for everyone involved.

By age ten, I knew all about problem feet and which arch supports and shoe "cookies," or inserts, could get me through a school day. Since sneakers were still out of the question, my participation in school sports was nil. Ballet and tap dancing lessons were also off-limits, and this deprived and absolutely ostracized me. I felt the pain, both physically and psychologically, of having abnormal feet. Until I was sixteen, I wore laced-up, brown, orthopedic oxfords. In a world where heels and T-straps reigned supreme, my feet immediately labeled me "misfit." Dating was difficult, to say the least.

After high school I began to take charge of my own two feet. While studying physical therapy in college, I finally learned how to rebel happily and comfortably in terms of footwear. My closet began to look like the average American college student's—except for an overabundance of heels, still my passion today! Though my foot problems hadn't gone away, I wore exactly what I wanted on my feet by learning how to shop for shoes, how to exercise the muscles of my legs and calves, how to stretch the ligaments of my feet, and which at-home foot-pampering programs worked best for my bunion and flat, wide feet which tired easily.

I discovered, too, that I was far from alone in my "foot focus." Millions of people like me suffered from regular foot aches and pains, most of us unnecessarily. I now know that eight out of ten foot problems can probably be prevented, and the rest can easily be cured. All those years of anguish were not necessary in my own case.

Out of school, working as a physical therapist with stroke victims, paraplegics, and amputees, many of them victims of the Vietnam war, I began to realize just how miraculous walking really is. I can remember watching policemen on the streets

walk easily along, mailmen coming up front steps, babies tod-
dling precariously, and ordinary men, women, and children
strolling, completely unaware of their center of gravity or of
how they managed to pick up each leg and put down one foot
after another. I realized how fortunate I was to have two legs,
bowed though they were, and two feet, no matter how wide,
flat, or bunioned. My serious interest in podiatry was born at
that point.

Except for the fact that I was a woman (most podiatrists are
men), as a physical therapist I was a perfect candidate for podiatry school. The way you move your entire body begins with
your feet. As a practicing podiatrist, I know the importance of
healthy feet, but as a woman, I understand the psychological
damage that can occur when a person is denied fashionable
shoes. Fortunately, if you know what to look for, you can find
a pair of shoes that are both comfortable and stylish, no matter
what type of feet you have.

I'm no longer upset or embarrassed by my feet when I go
shoe shopping. When I can't find the wider width I need in a
stylish pair of shoes, I simply tell the disdainful shoe salesman
that it is a shame that some shoe manufacturers refuse to ac-
knowledge feet that aren't A or B width. It's not my feet that
are the problem—for they are a pair among millions—but the
shoes themselves.

At the New York College of Podiatric Medicine, I was made
a scapegoat because the shoes I wore to class were the very kind
the professors cautioned patients against ever wearing. My flat
feet, wide width, bunions, and hammertoes made fine lecture
material, but I was sure the doctors were wrong. My shoes
weren't the cause of my foot ailments. The ailments came first.
What no one would believe was that my careful management
of my feet allowed me to wear delightful shoes and be the person
I always dreamed I could be.

You can have this freedom, too, if you take a long, hard look
at those feet of yours, find the pampering program that fits your
ache or ailment, and follow through on what I advise. I'll show
you how to assess your lifestyle, recognize your foot type, and

do easy exercises that can prevent problems from ever occurring. If you are a runner, a dancer, an athlete, or someone who simply dabbles in exercise, you will find practical solutions to your everyday foot problems. My guide to good foot products and some of my own recipes will serve you well. I'll give you an insider's look at the shoe industry and tell you how to find shoes that fit, when to shop for shoes, and everything you need to know about accessory footgear. Massage, reflexology, acupuncture, and the "sex life" of the lowly foot are other important aspects of this practical workbook.

In the days when my feet killed me this compendium of foot facts and fancies could have saved me much misery. I know it can help you.

Chapter 2
Why Your Feet Send Anguished Messages

In order to understand why your feet can hurt you, you need a clearer picture of this unmatched set of architectural wonders. (Unmatched? Yes, your feet were not created equal. Some individuals have feet which differ from each other by up to a full shoe size.)

Your feet are two of the most complexly engineered parts of your entire body. Each one has at least (experts disagree on the exact number) twenty-six bones, two very small bonelike sesamoids, fifty-six ligaments, thirty-eight muscles, and nerves and blood vessels too numerous to count. Take a look at your body, then glance down to the two feet that carry the weight of the rest of you. Marvelous, aren't they?

The twenty-six bones of each foot can be classified as seven tarsal bones, five metatarsals (the bones leading up to your five toes), and fourteen phalanges. Look at the illustration (Figure 2-1) to get a better idea of what I'm describing. These twenty-six major bones are cleverly and structurally arranged to permit the movements of the feet. Rotate your foot at the ankle. Bend your toes forward and then backward. Twist both feet inward so that you can see the soles. The precise and flexible arrange-

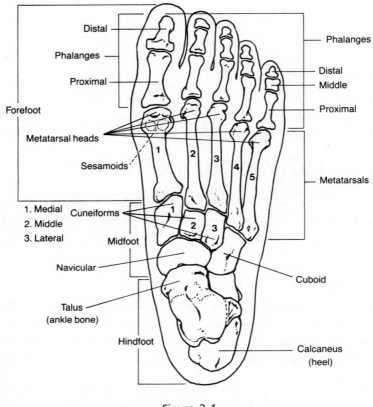

Figure 2-1
Bones of the foot (top view).

ment of your joints allows you to walk, run, jump, twist, or stand on the tips of your toes, "en pointe" if you are a ballerina.

Your foot can be subdivided into three sections: the hindfoot, the midfoot, the forefoot. The hindfoot consists simply of the talar joint, or ankle bone, and the heel bone, the calcaneus. The *subtalas* joint formed by these two bones is remarkable because of its unique flexibility. When twisting or moving your feet in a side-to-side rhythm, you may marvel at the beauty of this joint, but the next time you watch downhill skiing, you may see it as a biological miracle.

In your midfoot, there are five irregular bones called the tarsals, and together they form the arch. Your arch, whether it is high, medium, or so low that you are in the flat-footed category, is what provides the spring to your step. Inside the peak of this arch are three other bones called cuneiforms, and on the outside of the arch is the cuboid bone. Podiatrists usually refer to these midfoot bones as the *lesser tarsus* (Figure 2-2).

In your forefoot are five metatarsal bones and fourteen smaller

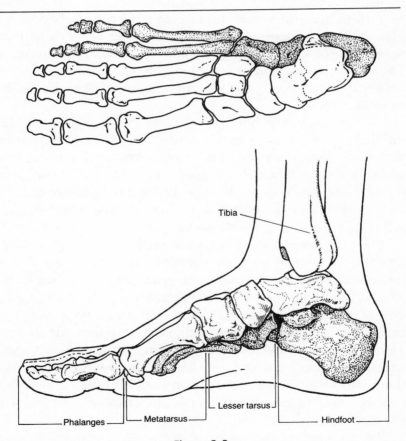

Figure 2-2
Functional units of the foot. The shaded areas provide support and the light areas are for shock absorption.

phalanges. The metatarsals bear the brunt of your weight as you walk and put pressure on the balls of your feet. Doctors used to believe that the body's weight was mainly supported in the heels or at the back of the foot, but now we know that 60 percent of the work is done by the balls of the feet. The metatarsals, as you may already have guessed or noticed in the illustration, continue up into your toes. The arch connecting the central part of your foot to your toes is known as the *metatarsal arch*. The smallest bones in your foot referred to as *sesamoids*, lie here, buried behind and beneath your big toe. Are they unimportant because of their minuscule size? Definitely not. People who have fractured or displaced either or both of these sesamoids soon experience acute pain and impaired movement. The sesamoids serve as a pulley system for some muscles, enabling them to move your foot up and down. They let the big toe move, too.

The five phalanges, or digits, or toes, are often referred to by number. Your big toe is number one, and you've got a number two, three, four, and five on each foot. Numbers two, three, four, and five toes each have three bones; your big toe has only two (besides the tiny sesamoids). The average little toe of today is smaller than its counterpart was 100 years ago. Why? Because we've been squeezing it into shoes.

While the bones and muscles are partly responsible for your ability to walk and stabilize yourself, you owe much to your ligaments. The longest ligament in your foot, the plantar fascia, which runs along the sole, is purported to be the strongest ligament in your entire body. When you stand, your weight is supported by the metatarsal arch, which flattens out slightly. That ligament along your sole is stretched just like a rubber band from your big toe to your heel. When you raise your foot, the ligament loosens and curves upward into your arch. When you step down again, the ligament absorbs most of the downward pressure.

The ligaments of the ankle are particularly vulnerable to injury. If these become torn or ruptured, they can take many months to heal.

The muscles of your feet are extremely important because they support these bony architectural devices which get you around. As important as the muscles themselves are the tendons which connect muscle to bone (Figure 2-3). Tendons can easily be ruptured, and I've seen many patients frustrated by the time

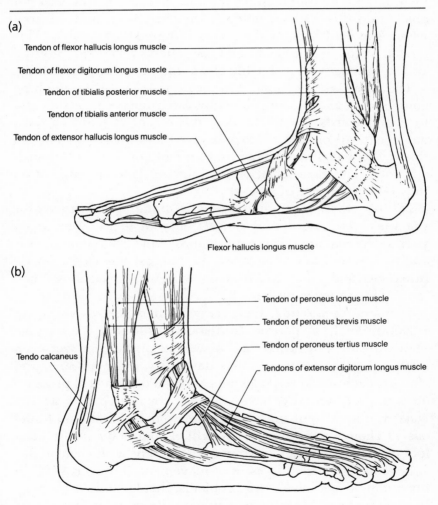

(a)

Tendon of flexor hallucis longus muscle

Tendon of flexor digitorum longus muscle

Tendon of tibialis posterior muscle

Tendon of tibialis anterior muscle

Tendon of extensor hallucis longus muscle

Flexor hallucis longus muscle

(b)

Tendo calcaneus

Tendon of peroneus longus muscle

Tendon of peroneus brevis muscle

Tendon of peroneus tertius muscle

Tendons of extensor digitorum longus muscle

Figure 2-3
(a) Medial aspect and (b) lateral aspect of the right foot.

it takes for a tendon to heal. Sometimes surgical repair is required. The largest and strongest tendon in your foot, the Achilles tendon, attaches your heel bone to the muscle which gives it mobility. Even if you aren't a jogger suffering from an overworked Achilles tendon, you have probably heard this name, taken from the Greek hero whose mother tried to make him invulnerable by dipping him into the river Styx. She was not able to do this without holding onto her baby, and the spot where she held him, at the ankle, remained vulnerable. This tendon at the back of your ankle is, in fact, very easily injured and can render you incapable of walking if seriously injured.

The complexity of your feet increases the chance of something going wrong and causing you pain. Environmental factors add to your hazards. Your feet were not meant to walk on hard pavement, strapped inside fashionable shoes with heels that can throw your weight onto a part of your foot not designed for such a burden. The ideal situation for your feet is to be barefoot on the yielding surface of a beach.

Falling, twisting, running, jumping, standing incorrectly for years, as well as dropping objects on your feet and stubbing your toes repeatedly can create foot problems. This general wear and tear as well as ordinary bruises, bumps, bad shoes, plastic rain boots, and nylon stockings make the work of walking much more difficult for your feet.

Speaking of walking, the average pair of feet travel up to 70,000 miles in a lifetime. Statisticians say that the average man walks 7 miles each day. A woman pushes her feet even further, logging up to 10 miles daily. If you are a 130-pound woman, each stride you take puts about 500 pounds of pressure on your feet. Actually, have you ever considered that as you walk, you aren't putting pressure on your two feet simultaneously? Though they share the weight of your body at rest, each foot carries the burden of your whole weight with each step.

Beyond the normal stresses of movement, however, some of my patients' feet have extra problems, thanks to their parents. For instance, people who have inherited very wide feet inevitably have difficulty finding shoes that fit properly and after many years end up with certain deformities, not because of their feet but because of their shoes. What I often see in these cases are bunions, blisters, painful corns, abrasions, and sometimes small ulcers between toes that are not able to stay straight inside tight shoes.

Another example of a predisposition for aching feet is the individual who inherits a high arch, or a cavus-type foot. What I have observed in these patients is that corns develop, sometimes at a very early age, across the tops of the toes; tendons grow painfully tight, prohibiting easy foot movement; toes contract or become bent in unhealthy directions; sometimes, the balls of cavus feet become so callused that it hurts to walk.

The person who inherits a low arch will develop a predisposition for bunions early in life, sometimes even before the bones are fully grown. (For more information about lifestyle, foot shape, and inevitable foot disorders, see "Observe Your Lifestyle.")

Still not convinced that your feet are worth paying attention to? Embarrassed by your feet? Leonardo da Vinci heralded the foot as "a masterpiece of engineering and a work of art." For centuries this often uncared-for part of our body structure has "nurtured custom, incited superstition, influenced fashion, and provided a universal means of expression through ceremony, dance, and sport," says Ruth Amdur Tanenhaus, organizer of a museum show called "The Great American Foot."

But, of course, you can't feel exultant about your feet if they are hurting you. As Abraham Lincoln said, "When my feet hurt, I can't think." So turn to the next section, designed to help you cure your feet of their aches as simply and as quickly as possible.

PART TWO
Foot-Pampering Programs

The first step toward pampered feet is to eliminate the specific problem putting you in pain. What I include in this second section are definitions, descriptions, and solutions for foot problems. Since most of my patients come into the office armed with questions, I use the simple question-and-answer format here too.

Chapter 3
The Callus

What Exactly Is a Callus?

A callus is an abnormal amount of dead, thickened skin which has built up because your body asked it to do so. Look at the bottom of your foot or along the outside of your big toe and you'll see that the ball of your foot and the end of your heel are the primary locations for this growth. The callus is probably thick, hard, yellowish-red in color, and just doesn't feel like your other skin. It is certainly not as soft or elastic as the skin on the top of your foot, is it?

You'll find calluses anywhere on your body wherever stress from excess pressure and friction occurs. Look at your elbows or the inside of your middle finger, the one you hold a pencil with, and you'll undoubtedly find some callused skin. I've known of gardeners who have extraordinary calluses on their hands due to the constant handling of garden tools.

But as long as a callus isn't troublesome, you can forget about it. A callus is there for protection. Your body produces it to cushion underlying bone from pressure at points where there is little fat or natural padding material.

Sometimes surprising occupations produce calluses. For instance, professional chauffeurs often develop unusually thick calluses on the bottoms of their feet from hitting the brake pedal and pushing down on the accelerator all day or all night long.

If Calluses Aren't Supposed to Be a Problem, Why Are They Painful Sometimes?

The extra pressure of a biomechanical problem may be to blame for your callus. For instance, if you aren't standing or walking properly, your feet may build up calluses in the weight-bearing areas, which can be quite painful. Sometimes a painful callus is caused by a malaligned bone or crooked toe. When one "toe bone" is lower than its neighbors, greater weight is placed on other points, and your body will try to compensate for your improper landing technique with a callus. But the callus will only work for a certain time before pain sets in. Then you'll have to do something to get rid of the excess callus and straighten out your biomechanical problem.

Painful calluses are most likely to be found on the balls of your feet, and they are being caused by abnormal motion in your forefoot. If you've got a low-arched foot, you are particularly prone to this. When too much callus builds up under the ball behind your big toe, you probably have a high-arched foot that isn't working perfectly.

How Do You Get Rid of a Bothersome Callus?

Start with your shoes. For instance, women who are high-heel fanatics are constantly shifting more of their weight onto metatarsal bones, causing increased stress on the balls of their feet and, therefore, excess callus formation. To ease the situation, they can switch back and forth between high- and low-heeled shoes. They should also look for high-heeled shoes with extra cushioning in the metatarsal area or have the shoe repair shop put extra foam cushioning in the forefoot of new shoes.

When Is a Painful Callus Problem Really Serious?

If you have what a professional podiatrist calls a "dropped metatarsal" bone or an intractable plantar keratosis, you've got trouble. By "dropped" I mean that one of the sesamoids behind your toes is much lower than the ones on either side of it. What can happen is that a thick, deep callus will build up to help even it all out, but in the process, such a callus can become excruciatingly painful. The calluses which come with hammer-toes and bunions—two problems you'll soon learn more about—can also be big problems.

The length of your metatarsal bones is instrumental in causing callus buildup. If the first bone is too short, you will definitely have callus forming under the second bone. And whenever the metatarsal bones are too long, you'll find thickened calluses beneath.

A relatively new way to treat calluses that are caused by a "dropped metatarsal" is through the use of collagen injections. The collagen acts as a cushion between the underside of the metatarsal and the outer skin. The benefits produced by the collagen injections, however, are not permanent since the collagen breaks down (much like the body's own connective tissue breaks down as we grow older) and the cushion disappears after about one year's time. Therefore, the collagen material needs to be reinjected on an annual basis to achieve maximum results from this technique.

Can Calluses Ever Be Mistaken for Something Else?

Yes. Sometimes calluses will form around warts or foreign bodies like splinters. I still remember the young woman who came to see me shortly after she had finished working on her hard-wood floors. She had been scraping, sanding, and staining, and it wasn't until the job was done that she noticed a strange-looking bumpy callus on the bottom of her heel. After trying to solve the mystery herself with a razor blade—never a good idea—she made an appointment to see me. The first thing we did in my office was talk about any change in her routine, and the story of her newly sanded floors came up. Then, after carefully cutting away the callused tissues, I found and removed a small wooden splinter. She was shocked. I wasn't. Her callus never came back.

Why Does a Pain-Free Callus Suddenly Become Painful?

When the dry, inelastic skin of a callus thickens too much, it causes constant irritation to the softer surrounding tissues. The nerve endings in the area react and send out pain signals. The spot soon becomes red and puffy and hurts even more. You may also feel a burning sensation, especially if you've been walking on hard pavements. The location of a callus is directly related to the presence or absence of pain. Obviously, if the callus is in a primary weight-bearing area, the ball of your foot, for instance, it will continue to thicken and may hurt if you ignore it. But since your entire foot is a weight-bearing extremity, it's not a good idea to let any calluses there go. You are simply asking for more calluses, and more problems. It can be a vicious circle.

How Do You Break the Bad Callus Cycle?

If you've got a very painful callus, go to a podiatrist and have it excised or cut away. If your callus is not making your life absolutely miserable, simply redistribute your weight on the area by using a callus pad or a moleskin, which is simply a soft cloth with one velvety side and one sticky side to hold it in place over your callus. If the callus isn't very thick and is causing you only minimal discomfort, you can treat it at home by soaking your feet and using an abrasive brush on the callus every day, followed by a cream to soften the callus. This daily brushing and creaming habit is a good one to adopt.

SUZANNE'S CALLUS SOLUTION

Patients with painful calluses smile when I first give them this recipe, but it works. Take five or six aspirin tablets, crush them into a powder, and mix with 1 tablespoon of water and 1 tablespoon of lemon juice. Make a paste, and apply it to all the hard-skin spots on your foot. Now, put your entire foot into a plastic bag, and wrap a warm towel around everything. The combination of the plastic and the warm towel will make the paste penetrate the hard skin. Sit still for at least ten minutes. Now, unwrap your foot and using a pumice stone (a rough-edged stone you can buy in a drug store for smoothing skin), scrub your foot, and use real rubbing action. All that dead, hard, callused skin should come loose and flake away easily.

One point you should remember about calluses is that the only real way to eliminate the painful ones and keep them from coming back is to correct the biomechanical problem which promoted their growth in the first place. Custom-made shoe inserts, called orthotics, can redistribute your weight inside your shoe and correct bony abnormalities. Orthotics are made of comfortable materials, and they should be a permanent shoe fixture for people with certain foot structures. For a perfectly fitting orthotic shoe insert, the podiatrist will make a cast of all or a part of your foot and then order the insert made to prescription. However, several manufacturing companies have jumped into the orthotics market, and sometimes one of their over-the-counter products will ease your pain. The next time you are in a store which carries foot products, take a long look at the assortment of inserts. In certain situations, such as the dropped metatarsal bone I mentioned before, surgery to correct the underlying bone deformity is the answer.

Calluses at the heel are caused by too much motion or rubbing. This type of callus is important to keep under control because it can easily become dried out and cracked, especially in menopausal women who have put on extra weight. Women with calluses on the back of their heels should avoid wearing open-backed shoes for awhile.

Are There Any Over-the-Counter Callus Medications That Really Work?

Some creams and ointments will eliminate your immediate problem, but their success is based on salicylic acid, a very caustic ingredient that can harm the surrounding skin. So be careful. To get rid of the callus forever, do something about the stress you are putting on the spot. Don't try to avoid the pain by walking lopsided, however. You could end up with an orthopedic problem instead of a simple callus condition.

Why Can't You Cut Away Your Own Callus?

Because it's very easy to cut more than the dead cells of the callus, and cutting live tissue will really hurt. When I remove a painful callus in my office, I soften it and then use a surgical blade to pare it down. It doesn't hurt because your callus has no nerve endings. Since it's dead tissue, it won't even bleed. If you try to perform this operation on yourself, from a contorted position, you may do a lot of harm. Please don't try; I've treated too many self-administered wounds.

Chapter 4
The Corn

When I think of a corn, in spite of all my years of podiatry, I still remember the television commercial that showed a throbbing corn miraculously pop out of the toe after the application of a certain remedy, to be gone forever. There was always something very satisfying about that image!

What Is a Corn?

A corn is a hard, thickened area of skin found on the top of, the tip of, or between your toes. It's very different from your normal skin and, like a corn kernel, it's round and yellow. If yours is reddish, you've got an inflamed corn. A corn has a central core which descends into your flesh in a cone-shaped point killing all the normal cells in its way. If you keep rubbing a corn against the side of a shoe, you speed up its growth by providing constant blood flow. More irritation means more blood circulation at the corn spot, and more corn cells growing.

Like calluses, corns are your body's response to friction and pressure. That corn is trying to protect both your skin and the bone beneath it from bruises and injuries.

Even though I've just stated that corns are usually yellow, or perhaps an inflamed shade of red, corns have been known to take on the color of a person's skin. I once treated a beautiful young black model who came to me because of ugly black dots on the tips of each of her toes. She was due to appear on film wearing sandals and was desperate to get rid of her strange crop of dots. She never considered that they could be corns. But corns they were.

Corns like the ones this model had are called *hard* because they are not like the *soft* ones found between your toes. Perspiration is what keeps this latter type soft.

Why Do You Get Corns While Others Simply Get Calluses?

Corns are confined to toes. (In fact soft corns almost always prefer a spot between your fourth and fifth little toes.) Calluses don't recognize such boundaries. If you have contracted or mis-shapen toes or bony abnormalities between the toes or if you regularly wear tight shoes, you're prone to painful corns. Toes should be able to lie flat within the confines of a shoe, though most of the time this isn't possible. Corns keep growing in response to the pressure put on them, and the bigger they get, the more painful they become.

How Do You Stop a Corn from Hurting?

The key to controlling the pain of a corn is to eliminate the pressure or friction coming from the improperly fitting shoe. Go out and buy shoes that fit comfortably even if it means a larger size or different style.

Your corn pain may be coming from a bursa, a fluid-filled sac that becomes inflamed and enlarged at the site between the bone and the corn. Bursas overlie and protect all the joints in your body. The overfilled bursa which may be beneath your painful corn would simply have been doing its job of protecting the bone, but the result is bursitis, an inflamed and swollen bursal sac.

One temporary pain relief measure I recommend is to soak your feet in a warm solution of epsom salts and water. You can find epsom salts in almost any drug store. This soaking will diminish the size of the bursal sac and take some pressure off the nearby sensory nerves. But a soak is only temporary. If you put on the same shoes that cramped your style in the first place, the bursa will soon swell back to its painful size. I remember a young woman who came to see me on a Thursday because of a large painful corn and its accompanying swollen bursa. I sent her home to soak her toes. After two hours with her feet in a tub, she was pain free. However, she went dancing on Friday night and wore her high-heeled shoes. Guess who called me on Saturday morning screaming about the pain?

If your corn is hard and there is no fluid sac, your pain can be reduced by getting rid of the hard skin. A podiatrist should do this for you, though. If you don't want to make a doctor's appointment right away, wear sandals that will put no pressure on your corn, or cut open an old pair of shoes to expose the corn. A piece of moleskin less than an inch in diameter can also help protect the corn from painful pressure.

Getting to the Root of Your Corn Problem

If you came to my office complaining about a painful corn, the first question I'd ask is, "When did it start to hurt?" Your answer would usually supply me with all the necessary information to get to the root of your problem. Most of the time, you'd have done something new—bought a new pair of shoes, joined an exercise class, gone to a dance, taken a long walk, started a new job. In this case, I might send you straight out to buy shoes with a wider toe box (the top portion of the shoe).

Sometimes, however, chronic corns are caused by a hammertoe condition which is discussed in Chapter 8, "The Hammertoe." Occasionally, flexible hammertoes can be corrected through a minor surgical procedure called a *tenotomy*. In this manner, recurring corns can be generally eliminated. With a more rigid hammertoe, several surgical procedures designed to alter the joint can be performed in a podiatrist's office under local anesthesia. Additionally, the collagen treatment, discussed earlier, brings relief to some corn sufferers and is the treatment of choice for those who are unable to undergo surgery.

How Can a Corn Appear Overnight?

It can't. But, if your corn is "acute" (which in this sense means that it has developed very recently, quickly, and with no prior history), I might remove the hard skin, place a piece of moleskin around the area, and recommend new shoes immediately. If the corn persists and is painful, an x-ray might be necessary.

When corns are due to an imbalance in the feet, I recommend orthotic inserts and order a plaster cast to be made of your feet to make the orthotic fit perfectly. When the corn is chronic, this often helps. Or, a podiatrist can also perform minimal incision surgery in the office and cut away the bony prominence making the corn such a nasty sight.

Can Corns Really Predict the Weather?

Yes, sort of. If the pressure in the atmosphere falls suddenly, the bursal sac near your corn can begin to rise. The extra fluid puts increased pressure on your sensory nerves and gives you pain. This is how a corn predicts the weather. But don't try to ask it for predictions. You'll only be disappointed.

Do Drug Store Corn Pads Ever Work?

No. Most over-the-counter corn removal remedies contain salicylic acid, a caustic substance that can cause blisters and infection, and may ruin the normal skin surrounding your corn. In fact, you might end up needing a podiatrist simply because of such a solution to your corn problem. If you want to treat your corn at home, soak your foot in epsom salts first, then apply moisturizing cream, cover the corn, and wrap the area in plastic for at least fifteen minutes. After you remove the plastic, use a pumice stone in a side-to-side motion to remove the hard corn skin. Please don't do surgery on yourself, however.

Is There a Particular Toe That Is Especially Prone to Hard Corns?

Yes. The fifth toe, or your little toe, is most definitely prone to corns. Generally, the toe rotates outward because of too much motion in the front of your foot. If you have too much pronation in the foot, and your arch has been flattening out in this process, your little toe hits against the top of your shoe a lot. This leads to corns. Sometimes the corn forms on the top of the toe, and sometimes it picks the side.

Chapter 5
The Blister

We all know what a blister is—this fluid-filled sac forms between the top layers of the skin and is probably the most annoying injury that a walker or jogger can experience.

What Causes a Blister?

Blisters are the result of friction between a shoe and the skin. Sometimes friction is so great that a blood blister, or hematoma, forms. A blister can be large or small, depending on how much friction is placed against the foot. We usually develop blisters on the ball of the foot, the back of the heel, or the tops of the toes. A blister is actually a protective device: it is the body's defense against the shearing forces of the shoe moving against the foot. Most blisters start off with redness and swelling, and a burning sensation. Sometimes your entire foot feels hot.

Can You Prevent Blisters?

Yes. The key is to find shoes that fit well. Next, properly fitting socks will prevent friction between the skin and the shoes, particularly when you are walking or jogging.

If you have bony toes or hammertoes, you might also try putting a bandage or moleskin over sensitive areas, to keep your shoes from rubbing against these areas. Finally, you can rub in petroleum jelly or any kind of emollient cream on areas you suspect might blister. Many athletes have found that putting lamb's wool over the tops of their toes helps prevent blisters. Foot powders also help reduce the frictional forces against the foot.

What Can You Do after the Blister Has Formed?

Sometimes, the best solution might simply be to leave the blister alone, particularly where a blister develops on a weight-bearing area (e.g., the bottom of the foot). However, the usual steps to take are to start by cleansing the skin with alcohol or an iodine solution like Betadine. Then use a sterile, sharp instrument and puncture the blister, making sure you leave the top part in place. Apply a topical antibiotic cream (Neosporin, Bacitracin, or Polysporin); then cover the blister with a bandage or a sterile piece of gauze or tape. The reason you want to keep the top of the blister intact is to avoid infection; the underlying skin is raw and sensitive. Often after a painless blister is punctured and the top skin and fluid are removed, the area becomes very painful, and sometimes even infected.

If you find that blisters seem to attack the sides of your toes all the time, particularly the large toe and the little toe, your shoes may be too narrow. If the blisters seem to form most often on the tops of the toes, your shoes may be too short. In either case, it is important to find out if your blisters are due to improper shoes or to faulty biomechanics of the foot. Sometimes a simple corrective device, such as an orthotic in your shoe, can help avoid the increased shearing forces on the foot, preventing blisters once and for all.

Chapter 6
A Gallery of Nail Disorders

Toenails protect the toes from injury. These hard, keratinous structures involve a plate, lunula, matrix, nail bed, nail fold, and cuticle (Figure 6-1).

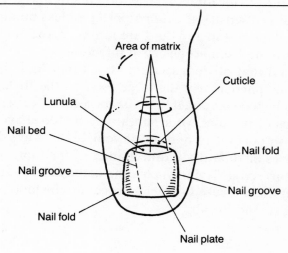

Figure 6-1
Parts of the nail and surrounding tissues.

Paronychia

Redness, swelling, and pain around the cuticle is usually due to trauma or excess manipulation of the skin during a pedicure. Once the skin is disturbed, it is easily infected with an organism such as *Staphylococcus pyogenes*.

How Can You Treat This at Home?

The best home remedy for a paronychia is to soak the feet in a solution of iodine (Betadine) and warm water for approximately fifteen minutes twice a day, if possible. Then, rub in a topical antibiotic cream. Alsó, avoid pedicures!

If after one or two days the pain continues to persist, it is time to see a podiatrist. Usually your doctor will cut into the paronychia and drain it. Then he or she will numb the toe with a local anesthetic and make a linear incision paralleling the infected nail fold. A culture is usually taken for laboratory analysis of the infecting organism. Finally, the infected area is coated with an iodine solution and covered with sterile gauze.

Onychomycosis (Ringworm)

You will first notice onychomycosis at the end of the nail, where it usually begins. Your nail will turn black or brown, and become thin and flaky-looking.

These fungal infections are very hard to treat—in fact, they may take one to two years to get under control. First, cut the nails as short as possible, and try to remove as much of the fungus as you can. Then you can apply antifungal agents. Potassium hydroxide and Whitfield's Ointment are very helpful. Use *oral* antifungal agents very carefully, and only under your doctor's supervision, because serious complications can occur. Griseofulvin, for example, can cause skin rashes, urticaria, angioneurotic edema, numbness in the hands and feet, nausea, vomiting, diarrhea, headaches, and granulocytopenia.

Black-and-Blue Nails

When your nail turns blackish blue, it is generally a sign of bleeding under the nail. This bleeding can be the result of a bruise, a blood disorder, or a vitamin C deficiency. The blood collected under the nail can sometimes be removed by drilling a small hole in the nail. Discoloration caused by a vitamin C deficiency can be reversed with the appropriate dosage of vitamin C.

Onychauxis

In onychauxis, the nail is very thick, particularly in older persons. It may even form a "ram's horn" shape, which is very hard to treat. The thickened nail can be caused by chronic dermatitis or some of the systemic disorders we experience as we grow older.

Filing down the nail with a rotary burr drill can help—this must be done by your physician. When the condition is very severe, the nail can be removed under local anesthesia.

Onycholysis

In onycholysis the nail plate begins separating from the nail bed, usually after repeated injury or immersion in harsh chemicals. In a few cases, a bony growth under the nail will force the nail up off the bed.

Effects of Disease on Nails

Infections such as syphilis and tuberculosis affect many body systems, including the nails. In early syphilis, the nails may shed. With tuberculosis, the nail bed may be very red and swollen. Leprosy, though rare, can cause complete changes in the nails or loss of them. Chronic arthritis can produce ridges in your nails. (For more information, see Chapter 10, "Arthritic Feet.") *Beau's lines* are transverse lines that give the nail an awkward, rough texture, and are due to interference with the production of keratin. Many diseases, including syphilis, tuberculosis, and some nervous disorders, can be the underlying problem.

Onychomadesis

In onychomadesis the nail separates from the nail bed, beginning at the bottom of the toenail. Often the old nail flakes off and a new nail grows in—this may take as long as six months. Trauma is the culprit here—I see this in many athletes, particularly joggers, who purchase new running shoes. The inflexibility of the new shoes causes them to abrade the toenails, in effect rubbing them off.

Toxic Causes

Many nail disorders are an overlooked "occupational hazard" brought on by toxic materials or drug sensitivities—when this occurs the nail plate separates from the nail bed.

Chapter 7
The Ingrown Toenail

Why Do Ingrown Toenails Hurt?

When the sides of your toenail—especially the big toe's nail—cut into the skin around the nail, the area can become very sensitive to pressure, especially from the side of a shoe. If the pressure continues because your shoes are tight around your toes, you'll end up with swelling, redness, and, of course, pain. What's happening is that the soft tissue on the side of your nail is reacting to the incurvating or ingrowing nail as if it were a foreign body.

What Made the Toenail Grow in the Wrong Direction?

Sometimes simply cutting your nail improperly can start the problem. Nails should always be cut straight across. If you cut a curve, or keep your nails too short, you create an ingrown toenail. Shoes that are too short or too tight for your toes can cause the nail to press into the sides of a toe.

How Serious Can an Ingrown Toenail Be?

A simple ingrown toenail is not a big problem. Often if you cut it properly, straight across, it will correct itself. But if you ignore a painful ingrown nail and let it become seriously infected, it can be very troublesome. Several patients have come to me only after they let their toe become red and swollen with pus. If your circulation is poor, you run the risk of gangrene. Sometimes a bloody growth, called a "proud flesh," builds up on the side of the nail. This inflamed soft tissue can become quite sensitive when it extends into the nail groove.

What Else Causes Nails to Ingrow so Painfully?

If your toenails do not naturally lie flat in their beds but appear more convex, or curved down, you are more likely to develop this condition. Faulty foot mechanics may also contribute. For instance, if you have flat feet, your big toe and forefoot are more likely to move incorrectly when you walk. A rolling motion of your toes will accentuate the pressure on the nails and create the perfect circumstances for toenail incurvation.

Can You Fix Your Own Ingrown Toenail?

Yes. First, avoid constant pressure on your poor toe. Cut out the portion of your shoe that presses on the toe or wear toeless sandals if you live in a warm climate. If there is an infection present, soak your foot in an iodine solution to reduce the inflammation. Next, cut or trim your nails and clean the nail grooves. Application of antibiotic cream is also helpful in reducing any inflammation.

If your pain persists, go to a doctor. Usually the physician will numb the nail with a local anesthetic at the base of your toe. When you can't feel anything, he or she will remove the portion of nail curving in and causing your pain. If your nail isn't infected, the doctor may decide to treat the root, or the matrix, of the toenail. Since this is more complicated, it might mean a stitch or two. If the ingrown toenail is infected, an antibiotic may be prescribed.

How Can You Avoid Ingrown Toenails?

Keep your toenails trimmed straight across and clean. Don't overtrim or interfere with the work your cuticles perform. If you pick at your toes too much, you make entries for bacteria. Wear shoes wide enough to give your toes breathing room, and stay away from tight pantyhose or socks.

BEWARE OF EXOTIC PEDICURES

One day a harried executive in suit and tie hobbled into my office wearing his bedroom slippers. He was quite a sight because he had even cut out a portion of the slipper to accommodate a very painful, swollen ingrown toenail. He told me he had been trying to doctor it himself for weeks using antibiotics. And when I questioned him about when it all began, I found out how fond he was of pedicures.

On a business trip to Japan not so long before, he had enjoyed placing his feet in the hands of an unusual pedicurist. Unfortunately, his right foot's big toenail hadn't been the same since. After taking a culture of the pus under the nail and removing a nail spicule, I prescribed another antibiotic for him. But I also warned him about letting a manicurist cut too deeply into any nail groove in the future. This poor man had to return to my office twice more before he could wear his shoes comfortably.

Chapter 8
The Hammertoe

The twisted hammertoe makes me angry when I consider what it does to a set of straight and narrow phalanges. Just because you've asked the joint in one of your middle toes to bend to fit the space allotted doesn't mean you want it to stay that way forever.

Why Is a Hammertoe So Called?

A hammertoe is not caused by a hammer dropping onto your toe. It is a permanent deformity of one of your middle toes—probably the big toe's neighbor—in which the joint has become bent up and twisted. It looks like the small hammer inside the workings of a piano. "Aha!" you say. "Who was the fool who named a misshapen toe after a piano?" I don't know, but I do know that if the bent toe joint is the one near the tip as opposed to the inside joint, it's called a *mallet toe*.

Why Do You, in Particular, Have to Have a Hammertoe?

Most hammertoes are the result of heredity. If you have a high-arched foot like your mother or father before you, you are more likely to end up nursing a hammertoe through life. Or if your second toe is exceptionally long even if no one else in your family can brag of this eccentricity, you may force it into the permanently bent, hammertoed condition, especially if you like pointy-toed cowboy boots or high heels.

There are several other congenital foot shapes that can put you in hammertoe danger. A pronated foot (and *pronated* simply means you have an arch which sags) will cause you to have excessive motion in your forefoot, which will make your big toe turn in toward its neighbor and may eventually send that neighbor's joint up into a bend, giving you the unfortunate hammertoe.

Hammertoes may also come from injuries. If you have damaged or dislocated any of your metatarsal bones, this can set up a dangerous cycle for your ligaments. Loose or altered ligaments can cramp your toes into permanent bends and twists.

Shoes don't help your hammertoe situation either, as I have mentioned. For example, if you continually squeeze into shoes that are too short for your toes, they are going to curl up to fit the space they're allotted. Years of squeezing can leave you with a permanently unsightly and twisted toe.

Do Hammertoes Hurt?

Not necessarily. The hammertoe itself is painless. When your hammertoe hurts, it is because it has been rubbing against something which has aggravated a nearby bursal sac. It can be an excruciating experience.

How Do You Get It to Stop Hurting?

Cover the hammertoe with a pad, such as a corn pad, or use lamb's wool or a bandage to alleviate the pressure on it. You might also want to examine your old shoes for a pair that you wouldn't mind cutting open. Any kind of shield, padding, or opening will relieve the pain temporarily.

What Can a Podiatrist Do?

On your first visit to my office, I would take an x-ray to see just how severely the toe was deformed. Sometimes a joint has become fused, or permanently stuck. If the tissue all around is inflamed from bursitis, I might suggest minor surgery. If you are an active individual, not willing to confine yourself due to recurring disability from a sore toe, surgery is often your best bet.

Correcting a flexible hammertoe surgically is not difficult. A flexible hammertoe is one that can be manually straightened out by putting pressure on the top to force it to lie flat. In fact, I classify it as a minor surgery. The procedure involves lengthening the tendons along the top of your toes through a very small incision. The incision is so small, you don't even need stitches, but when this stiffened tendon is relaxed, you can usually begin to use your toe joint again.

Another type of hammertoe surgery can be performed when the hammertoe is more rigid. It involves actually removing the toe joint. This is called *arthroplasty*, and sometimes it is the only option. It can be done under local anesthesia. You will end up with a shorter toe and a scar, but your pain will be permanently eliminated, and that may be worth it.

How Long Is the Recovery Period after Hammertoe Surgery?

If you have had the tendons relaxed, you will be back in the swing of things fairly rapidly. If no other major health problems are interfering, two weeks should see you through the recovery. If you have had arthroplasty, it may take longer. But your own doctor will predict your personal recovery time.

Chapter 9
The Bunion

When patients show me their sore, strangled toes and the painful, twisted knob of a bunion on the side, I can't help sympathizing with these patients, who are in pain with every step.

What Is a Bunion All About?

A bunion is one of the most distressing problems that your big toe can have. Not only is it painful, it is ugly and can turn shoes into torture chambers. I use the plural for shoes here, because bunions often come in pairs. If your right toe has one, the left is probably not far behind. Sometimes bunions make a forefoot so wide that wearing normal shoes is impossible, and I don't know anyone who would choose to spend his or her life with a big bunion exposed in sandals or padded in a pair of molded orthopedic shoes. What punishment the poor foot has to endure.

Sometimes after carefully examining a patient's foot, I look at the shoe as well. The shoe is almost always distorted and ruined by the bunion formation. Nothing seems to conceal a bunion.

This bony bump on the outside edge of your big toe is a form of arthritis. It indicates that degenerative changes are taking place in the bone beneath. If you were able to look inside your toe under a microscope, you would see "pock-marked," yellowing cartilage, and an equally distressing picture of the accompanying bone.

If you've got such a lump, you can usually, but not always, count on having a deviation of the big toe called *hallux abducto valgus*. *Hallux* means "great toe," *abducto* means "outward," and the *valgus* indicates an abnormal turning away. In fact, the bunion may be causing your first toe to push inward against your second toe and create a hammertoe. I've seen big toes so deviated from normal that their toenails couldn't be seen from above. This deformity will give you a very wide foot and cause sagging of the arch because of the way your toe is pulling everything out of shape. In severe cases of hallux abducto valgus, you can't stand up for very long without losing your balance, because your feet aren't able to support or balance your body properly.

Not all bunions result in complete swinging-in of the big toe. There are simple bunions which appear on the side of a straight big toe and others on the top of the big toe joint, as opposed to the side. Bunions have also been known to plague little toes, but these are often called "bunionettes" or "tailor's bunions."

What Makes a Bunion Hurt So Much?

When your bunion is accompanied by bursitis, an inflammation of the bursal sac beneath and next to the bone, you are in trouble. As I've mentioned, bursas swell and become painful with too much friction. Such bursas are called *adventitious* because they have formed in response to trauma. *Adventitious* has the sense of "not inherent," and "in an unusual place."

THE FINGER TEST

Here is a quick and easy test to let you know if you have bursitis at your bunion site: (1) Push down on the bump. Does a whitish area appear when you press it? (2) Release. Does the area turn red? If so, you may have bursitis.

Ordinarily, a bursa becomes redder and more swollen as the bunion gets larger and interferes with the movement of the bone beneath. Warmth is another sign of the inflammation.

What If Your Twisted Big Toe Is Stiff as Well as Sore?

Sometimes a turned-in big toe with a bunion is also afflicted with what podiatrists call *hallux limitus*. *Limitus* indicates the great toe's restricted ability to move up and down. The pain in this case comes not only from the bunion, which may or may not be inflamed, but also from the rigidity of the toe. Rigidity of the toe generally occurs as a result of arthritic changes in the first metatarsal phalangeal joint (see Chapter 10, "Arthritic Feet"). Pain is expressed when the metatarsal head rubs against the base of the first phalanx. Depending on how limited the range of motion is in your joint, all of your weight can be transferred onto the ball of your foot and the second metatarsal bone. Hallux limitus is usually found only in older people.

Who Can You Blame for Your Bunion?

Like many other foot problems, bunions are hereditary. If you ask parents and grandparents to expose their feet, you'll soon discover similarities to your own. Certain inherited foot structures will make you more susceptible to bunions, for instance, pronated feet (sagging arches).

Shoes may contribute to bunions, but they are never the only cause. Studies have shown that even people who never wear shoes—who live on tropical islands, for example—are plagued by bunions.

Why Do All the Women in Your Family Have Bunions and Not the Men?

Statistics show that women have a much greater chance of developing bunions. There is no explanation for this cruel fact of life. Women's shoes are often blamed, but they alone cannot account for the high numbers. The sex differences which show themselves in foot shape (i.e., lighter bone structure) and the hormonal differences between men and women could be the explanation.

What Can You Do for an Inflamed Bunion Late on a Saturday Night?

If there is no chance of getting professional help immediately, the best treatment is the simplest: ice. Apply ice packs to your bunion for fifteen minutes, three or four times a day, to reduce the acute inflammation. Put your foot in a tub of ice if you must, but cool it down.

Next, reduce the amount of pressure on the area by wearing a very wide shoe, a sandal, or a sneaker with a hole cut out to accommodate the bunion. I also suggest that patients create their own bunion pads by cutting moleskin in a doughnut shape or using shapes of foam rubber. For more chronic inflammation, I advise soaking the area for fifteen minutes in a mixture consisting of one cup of vinegar for every gallon of warm water. The vinegar is excellent for helping to reduce inflammation and alleviate pain.

Any kind of analgesic such as aspirin is good, too. When you get to a doctor, ask about physical therapy using ultrasound (a form of deep heat transmitted by a pulsating crystal), electrogalvanic stimulation, paraffin baths, or whirpool massage. Each of these treatments has been successful with my patients.

An orthotic shoe insert, special insoles, or arch supports can sometimes change the way you walk and take pressure off your sore big toe. In many cases, orthotics work miracles for people in bunion pain, and they can keep a bunion from ever getting out of hand.

But How Do You Permanently Get Rid of a Bunion?

You've probably noticed by now that I've been talking about eradicating your bunion pain, not your bunion itself. Only surgery can clear up your problem once and for all.

There are several different surgical procedures, but in most cases they are done on an ambulatory basis. You walk into the doctor's office and walk out slowly. There is no need for overnight hospitalization for the average person. Some bunion procedures don't even require stitches after a minimal incision, instead, a special type of adhesive strip is used called a butterfly closure.

What Do You Need to Know about Bunion Surgery?

Even though every patient is slightly different and your doctor should suggest the procedure best for you, it is helpful to know a few of the various techniques, if only to enable you to ask the right questions.

A Simple Bunionectomy In this procedure, only the bump is removed, and some of the soft tissue in the toe is repaired. The best candidates are patients whose toes are still fairly straight. If you opt for a simple bunionectomy and you also have a deviated great toe, in the long run you could develop another bunion.

The Fractured Bone Bunionectomy When you have a deviated toe as well as a bunion, a podiatrist may choose to break and realign the toe and shave off the bunion at the same time; this technique is known as an akin procedure. Another procedure, the Austin or Mitchell bunionectomy, involves the fracture and realignment of the first metatarsal head and excision of the bunion. There are many variations of this approach, so if a doctor starts talking about breaking your toes to get rid of your bunions, don't be surprised.

The Keller Bunionectomy   Named after the surgeon who designed the procedure, a Keller bunionectomy involves the removal of a small portion of the bone or joint from the base of your big toe. This is not a procedure I usually recommend for a young person, because it can make the toe stiff and shorten it. However, on occasion, an implant can correct the stiffness.

The Radical Bunionectomy   A "radical" procedure simply means that you are having your bunion removed, with the toe surgically fractured and realigned using internal wires or pins. The pins come out after the bone has healed properly.

When Does Bunion Surgery Require Hospitalization?

After performing many types of bunionectomies in the hospital, I have concluded that my patients recuperate faster when they choose office surgery. Unless you have a history of diabetes or some serious medical complication, a podiatrist can treat you on a Friday, send you home to stay off your feet for several days or a week, and bill you for far less than the more involved overnight hospital stay would cost.

Whatever procedure you choose, pick a doctor in whom you can have confidence, someone who will answer each of your questions without making you feel foolish.

What Kind of Complications Does Bunion Surgery Entail?

No surgery is utterly without complications, but foot surgery has come a long way in recent years because of the acceptance of minimal incision procedures. (See "Foot Surgery" below.) Whether your doctor chooses a simple bunionectomy or a radical procedure, it is going to be several months before normal shoes feel good on your feet. So be patient. If you must undergo surgical fractures, it can take six to eight weeks for the bone to heal. By not scheduling any skiing trips or running in the sand, you'll speed up the healing process. Staying off your feet keeps the swelling down.

Will Surgery Hurt More than the Bunion Itself?

No. My patients tell me that having bunion surgery is similar to going to the dentist. They know the work is being done but they don't feel any pain during the procedure. And I almost always prescribe an analgesic such as Empirin with Codeine or just aspirin to alleviate minor discomfort that one might experience from any skin opening. Normally, the surgical wound will heal completely within 14 days. If I've inserted wires or pins, they come out after four weeks. During healing, cutouts in shoes or surgical slippers are recommended, but it's not long— six to eight weeks, for instnce—before you are back in fashionable shoes and feeling good in them for what may be the first time in years.

TO IMPROVE A TENNIS GAME

Several months ago, a very sophisticated international banker came to me complaining of a very painful bunion. It had gotten so out of hand, he had even begun to take his shoe off underneath the conference table. He was also upset that it was spoiling his tennis game. Six months after I removed the bunion, I saw him at an indoor court in the middle of a very aggressive tennis game. I was certain he was pain free when I watched him destroy his opponent 6–1, 6–2, 6–0.

Can You Have Your Bunion Removed with Microsurgery?

No. Microsurgery involves the use of a microscope during surgery. When a doctor is reattaching a nerve, muscle, tendon, or vein, microscopes are generally employed. But when a podiatrist performs minimal incision surgery, a microscope is not needed.

Are Lasers Ever Used to Remove Bunions?

No. A laser can only be used to remove soft tissue. It can't cut through bone.

Will You Have Scars after Bunion Surgery?

No corrective procedure can make your foot appear as though surgery was never performed; nor can I ever guarantee a bunion patient complete range of motion after surgery. The surgical procedure will be influenced by your genes, your body's biochemistry and healing process, the way you walk, and the kind of shoes you wear. Even in individuals who have excellent results, a scar can remain. Remember that scars eventually fade and that plastic surgery can offer solace to some individuals.

FOOT SURGERY: A PATIENT'S GUIDE

Many years ago, a bunion, a hammertoe, or a bony enlargement on your foot would send you straight to the hospital or the orthopedist's office. An orthopedist is a doctor with a medical degree who specializes in the treatment of bones.

Podiatrists today are highly trained surgeons who specialize in the treatment of the foot. The ambulatory surgery they perform on a regular basis is as close to pain free as you can imagine. Many podiatrists call it painless.

Can You Describe a Typical Ambulatory Procedure?
Let's take a bunionectomy. To remove a simple bunion, the foot is scrubbed thoroughly with surgical soap and painted with iodine. A local anesthetic is injected around the surgical site. This is the same

kind of anesthesia your dentist uses. A linear incision is made in the skin. You don't feel this cut, because the area is numb. After the soft tissue is gently pulled from the underlying bone, an instrument is used to remove the bony bump. Then any soft tissue abnormalities or contractions are corrected using a sewing material that will be absorbed and metabolized by your body. The skin is then closed with stitches, or sutures, that will come out in 14 days, and bandaged with gauze and any other materials necessary to protect the surgical site.

What are the Common Postoperative Precautions?
You will be asked to avoid getting your foot wet for two full weeks, until the sutures are removed. I usually recommend that patients wear a plastic bag on their foot when they bathe or shower.

Is This Type of Surgery Replacing the Hospital Orthopedic Procedures?
For many foot problems, ambulatory, in-office surgery is an alternative. It is not an option for serious reconstruction work. It is ideal when you need to get rid of a bony formation or straighten a deviated big toe.

Reconstructive surgery is indicated when the foot has been severely injured or is malformed because of disease or congenital abnormality. This type of procedure almost always requires general anesthesia and extensive hospitalization.

What Exactly Is Minimal Incision Surgery?
Minimal incision surgery has become very popular in recent years because it is office surgery and entails only a small incision in your foot. The podiatrist uses a special burr, or circular drill (like the ones in your dentist's office), to make a small opening, perhaps ½ inch, in the surface of the skin. Another burr is placed under the skin at the site of the bony enlargement and is used to carefully smoothe down the deformity. Without being able to see it, the surgeon can explore the entire bunion. To remove all the tiny pieces of chipped bone takes time and requires precise work.

My Friend Had Ambulatory Foot Surgery to Remove a Bunion and Then It Came Back. Why?

Statistics show that one out of every fifty foot conditions that require surgery do return. But in the case of a bunion, sometimes what appears to be a bunion is simply swelled soft tissue. This lump will eventually disappear, but it may take up to a year. This is because it is impractical to immobilize the foot and isolate it from gravitational forces for long periods of time.

In addition, due to the positioning of the tiny sesamoid bones underneath the big toe (first metatarsal), in some feet it is virtually impossible to remove all the bony enlargement of a bunion without displacing these tiny bones. Walking would be painful or perhaps even impossible without the sesamoid bones. The podiatric surgeon has to use fine judgment about just how much of the extra bone to remove. The appearance of your foot is not the only factor the podiatric surgeon must consider; the sesamoid factor is a critical one.

Chapter 10
Arthritic Feet

Bunions are only one of the ways arthritis can show itself in your feet. Pain in the soles of your feet, gout in your big toe, and swollen ankles are among the other manifestations. When I realize that arthritis is responsible for their problems, I send patients along to a rheumatologist, a specialist in treating arthritic conditions. Dr. Michael J. Colin is a rheumatologist in New York City, and I've asked him to answer the most common questions concerning arthritis and feet.

How Does Arthritis Affect Your Feet?

Arthritis is an inflammation of the cartilage and lining of your joints. Since your feet contain cartilage as well as some key joints, they are especially susceptible to arthritis pain. Pain is the number one symptom to watch for.

What Happens When Arthritis Begins?

If for some reason the number of synovial cells which line a joint increases, the joint can become enlarged and thickened.

Too much fluid is produced by the cells, and it accumulates in the tissues, causing the joint to swell. Your joint or joints may feel swollen, spongy, soft, hard, or tender. The pain will vary, depending on the type of arthritis.

The expanding synovium (layer of synovial cells) also causes other problems, including inflammation. Again, the degree of pain and inflammation depends on the type of arthritis that is present. Some people have chronic arthritis that lasts for years, while others have short, mild episodes.

It's important to know that whatever type you have, if the inflammation isn't treated, both cartilage and bone usually will be damaged. Once the damage is done, it is irreversible. It becomes much harder to move your joints, and pain can increase. For this reason, treatment is essential and should be immediate. Treatment is aimed at preventing progression of your arthritis and destruction of the joint.

Cartilage: The Critical Connection

Normal cartilage acts as a buffer between bones. Its spongy structure holds substances that make it strong and resilient. Normal cartilage can withstand tremendous forces and lasts for decades. Sometimes, however, the chemical composition changes, and the cartilage loses its natural strength. It may become dry, crack, and split, fissuring down to the bone. The cells of the cartilage then wear away, and the bone may be exposed. You may then feel pain. What happens next is that excess fluid gathers in the joint. This is the process that will lead to arthritis.

Why Is Arthritis So Painful?

Arthritis pain is caused by chemicals in the joint that control inflammation. These chemical mediators are released by the cells of the synovium and certain white blood cells. The white blood cells are responsible for the acute and chronic inflammation of arthritis. Certain chemicals that are released from the white blood cells, called prostaglandins, are very powerful and can cause pain. Other chemicals make blood vessels expand, and cause you even more pain. Still other chemicals, called enzymes, may damage the joint tissue if they are allowed to remain in the joint for too long.

In the later stages of the disease, the damage which has been done to the cartilage and bone causes more chronic pain because the abnormal cartilage and exposed bone are constantly rubbing.

Pain is very subjective, and it is always difficult for a physician to judge how much you are experiencing. Rheumatologists like me are trained to evaluate the entire clinical situation and to recognize and deal with all degrees of pain.

Rheumatoid Arthritis

Rheumatoid arthritis, or RA, is a specific disease of the synovium. It usually begins very gradually, affecting one joint, then another and another. It can attack any joint. The small joints of the feet, the metatarsal joints, and the toes are common targets. The ankle and the small joints in the middle of your foot are often involved as well. The symptoms of RA are swelling, pain, and warmth.

Who Gets Rheumatoid Arthritis?

Rheumatoid arthritis is three to four times more common in women than men, and usually strikes first in early middle age, in the thirties and forties. A second peak occurs in the seventies. (RA can also occur in children and young adults. For the most part, the symptoms and courses of juvenile and adult forms of rheumatoid arthritis are the same.)

Since RA starts insidiously, you may simply notice aches and pains in a few joints. More joints become involved, the pain gets worse, and swelling soon follows. Often the joints feel warm to the touch. In more severe cases, walking, working, or doing daily chores becomes burdensome. Many persons notice that they tire easily, but sleep is interrupted by pain. The continual pain brings its own set of problems, including depression and time lost from work. At its worst, rheumatoid arthritis results in permanent disability.

The devastating effects of RA can be minimized with proper treatment, and you should be aware that no more than 5 percent of persons with RA actually develop "crippling arthritis" requiring walking aids or a wheelchair. The overwhelming majority do very well.

HOW DOES IT FEEL?

Ann is a forty-three-year-old housewife whose first symptom was pain in her feet. At first, the bottoms of her feet hurt at the end of the day. Then she noticed she had increasing difficulty walking when doing her shopping and daily chores. Her toes, the tops of her feet, and her ankles began to swell. The pain worsened, and she became frightened. She was tired in the afternoons and needed a nap to get through the day. Now other joints began to ache and swell as well. She tossed and turned at night, unable to get a good night's sleep.

After three weeks of such symptoms, Ann came to see me. When I examined her, I found many swollen, warm, tender joints in the feet, ankles, and hands. The balls of her feet were particularly tender and painful. A blood test showed that she had elevated rheumatoid factor (a positive sign of RA), and a very high sedimentation rate, which is a way of measuring the degree of inflammation of the joints. She was also anemic.

After discussing her illness and possible ways of treating it, she and I decided upon a course of nonsteroidal anti-inflammatory agents and gold injections. She learned that she could expect to be more tired, stiffer, and to continue to have pain until the disease was under control. An afternoon nap was prescribed, along with vitamins, a balanced diet, and medication. While RA wasn't anything Ann would have wished for, her arthritis was under control.

Gout: Not Just a King's Ransom

Gout has been around for centuries; in fact, it was first described by Greek and Roman physicians. Gout was known to Hippocrates (5th century B.C.) and Galen (129–199 A.D.). The fifth century Byzantine physicians treated gout with colchicine, the drug that is *still* used for joint pain. Gout gained notoriety during the middle ages, when King Henry VIII of England was a sufferer. Gout became known as the "disease of the wealthy," probably partly because of its association with the fatty diets and alcohol that only the rich could regularly afford.

Gout is still common today. It can be an inherited condition, and is more frequently found in men than women; women usually don't get attacks until after menopause, which may be due to the protective effects of estrogen. In men gout usually begins in the thirties and forties. Generally it is caused by an accumulation of uric acid crystals in the joint. Gout may be aggravated by an overly rich diet.

A MEAL WITH A REAL PRICE

Early one Sunday morning, a fifty-two-year-old stockbroker awoke with an extremely painful, red, and swollen left big toe. The night before, he had enjoyed a full-course French dinner of pâté, filet mignon with brandied cream sauce, and three glasses of wine, followed by chocolate mousse and a liqueur.

Now he lay in bed in agony, unable to stand even the weight of the sheet on his big toe. He had never experienced anything this painful before. He could not put on his shoe; walking was nearly impossible, and thus he stayed in bed the rest of the day.

On Monday morning he hopped into my office on his one good foot; with a slipper on his other foot cut out at the toe to make room for his throbbing big toe. When I examined him, I found mildly elevated blood pressure and the swollen, red, and tender left toe. The toe was especially painful on the inside.

The findings pointed to a classic case of acute gouty arthritis. I removed a small amount of fluid from his painful joint and examined it under the microscope, looking for quantities of uric acid crystals, which would confirm the diagnosis. They were there!

The patient was shocked. I prescribed indomethacin (Indocin) after meals and at bedtime. By the next morning, he was able to put his shoe on and go to work. He still had some pain, but by the fifth day of treatment the attack was completely over. A week later, when he came in for follow-up blood and urinary tests, the uric acid levels were normal. What the stockbroker was beginning to learn and what I try to teach all my patients is that they can prevent future attacks by monitoring what they eat and avoiding foods that give them trouble.

Gout is sudden and painful. It has a real predilection for the first joint of the big toe. (This is the place where bunions so often develop.) An attack may be so awful that you can't put your shoe on or stand anything touching your toe.

What Is the Significance of Uric Acid?

The extreme inflammation in gout is caused by accumulation of thousands of uric acid crystals in the joint. These microscopic crystals are attacked as foreign bodies by the white blood cells. The white blood cells then attract more white blood cells, which further fuels the fires of inflammation. The process is so severe that it can mimic an infection. In fact, some attacks of gouty arthritis are misdiagnosed as infections and treated with antibiotics. The true diagnosis of gout can always be established by an examination of joint fluid under the microscope.

PAIN AND A PINK EYE

Ben, a twenty-six-year-old man, developed pain and burning on urination, which finally cleared up after ten days. A few days later he noticed pain and swelling in the fourth toe of his right foot, the second toe of his left foot, and pain and redness behind both heels. Later, his left knee swelled up and walking became almost impossible. He couldn't even get his shoes on because of his painful heels. He limped into my office for help.

When I examined him, I found his left eye showed conjunctivitis (pink eye). His left knee was very swollen, warm to the touch, and painful to move. The fourth left toe and second right toe were both red and sausage-shaped, with very tender, painful joints. His Achilles tendons were swollen and thickened at their attachment to the heel bone. Ben's physical examination and blood tests, along with the history, were clear-cut evidence of Reiter's syndrome, which is a form of reactive arthritis. I prescribed indomethacin therapy, and he had an excellent response.

Ben's problem was related to a group of arthritic conditions similar to RA that develop after an infection. Such infections may occur in the bowel, associated with acute diarrhea, or, as in Ben's case, in the urinary tract, causing urethritis, or inflammation of the urethra. The inflections can follow bacterial dysentery caused by organisms such as *Shigella* or, less commonly, *Salmonella.* Urethritis is marked by pain or burning during urination. When urethritis, arthritis, and conjunctivitis, or pink eye, are present, the disease is called *Reiter's syndrome.* While the symptoms are clear in men, the disease may go unsuspected in women, for there are far fewer (or no) symptoms. Children and teenagers may also be affected.

When this type of arthritis involves the feet, it can attack the ankle joints, the small joints of the toes, the ligaments attached to the undersurface of the heel, and the Achilles tendon. It may affect only one or two joints of the foot and can also affect the arms. When the Achilles tendon and its surrounding soft tissues are involved, it is again most likely Reiter's syndrome.

Arthritis and Colitis

Arthritis may develop with colitis or ileitis in almost any joint, frequently the ankles and joints of the toes. This conjunction is more likely when inflammatory bowel disease is active and flaring. It may seem hard to make the association between bowel disease and arthritic symptoms, since they are so vastly different, but when bowel disease is well controlled by medication, joint pain is much less severe. Therefore if you are troubled with bowel disease, it is important to keep it under control to successfully treat and avert any accompanying arthritis.

Psoriatic Arthritis

Psoriasis is a common dermatological problem. The scaly plaques of psoriasis usually affect the scalp, elbows, or knees, but can also appear in a more widespread form. If you scratch these scales, the skin will flake off, and there will be bleeding at the base. Fewer than 5 percent of patients will develop arthritis along with psoriasis. When they do, arthritis will often involve the feet, affecting the last joints of the toes, the ankle, and other foot joints. Unlike RA, usually only one side of the body is affected.

If you have psoriasis, it is important that it be kept under control. Because the lesions may occur in unsuspected places, the psoriasis may be a hidden cause of arthritis.

Osteoarthritis

Another common disorder, particularly in older persons, is osteoarthritis, which is characterized by changes in the joint cartilage. The chemical changes we mentioned earlier that lead to the breakdown of cartilage seem to occur with age and with wear and tear. Pain begins to occur each time you move, and sometimes fluid accumulates in the joints.

Osteoarthritis can follow sudden or severe injury to the joint or more gradual, repeated trauma. The small joints in the toes, the ankle joints, and the joints in the middle of the foot are most commonly affected. Hammertoes and bunions may eventually lead to osteoarthritis of the metatarsal joints—particularly if these joints are forced down to the sole and thus exposed to pressure and trauma. For the many people who have bunions and hammertoes, the overall risk of osteoarthritis is even higher. If you find you have pain while walking, you should seek medical attention.

Joint Infections

Occasionally a bacterium or virus gets into a joint and starts an infection. When it's not treated, infection can cause severe, painful arthritis. This may also develop in association with a viral infection elsewhere, such as in the upper respiratory tract. Usually only one joint will be affected.

CHILLS IN THE NIGHT

Jane is a sexually active college student who developed fever and chills one night. The next morning, she found three small, tender, round bumps—two on her toes and one on a finger. Then she had trouble bending and straightening her fingers and toes. Her ankle began to swell and became painful. She was definitely worried.

While I was taking her medical history, she mentioned that she was having a slightly greater than usual vaginal discharge. Her temperature was 100.6 degrees F. I put her in the hospital.

After removing a little fluid from her ankle with a needle and syringe, and two days of analysis, I discovered that the cause of her infection was gonorrhea. A few days of treatment with penicillin helped her ankle and, after a week she was discharged from the hospital. She continued to take oral antibiotics at home, however.

How Is Arthritis Linked to Gonorrhea?

Gonorrhea is very common in young adults like Jane. Women may have a virtually symptom-free case of gonorrhea that finally shows up in the joints and tendons of the feet.

Other organisms, such as streptococci, pneumococci (as in

pneumonia), and staphylococci ("staff infections"), can also lead to joint infections in your feet. The first signs will be fever and chills; then a joint will become swollen and painful.

For all cases of bacterial infection, taking a sample of fluid from the swollen joint and asking a laboratory to identify the organism is the first step in treatment. Antibiotics will then eradicate the infection and cure the arthritis.

How Do You Treat Arthritis?

If you came to my office for treatment, the first thing I would do is listen to your description of your symptoms. Questions about your symptoms, some of which might seem totally unrelated to arthritis, are nonetheless very important.

Next, I would perform a complete physical examination. I'd test all your joints (not just those of your feet), your muscles, your reflexes, your overall strength, and examine your spine. I might also order an x-ray of your joints. Blood tests are usually necessary as well.

The most important step is to find the treatment that will help you feel better. The types of treatment available today are far more diverse and much more effective than ever before. If you have rheumatoid arthritis, we will try to make the disease go into remission, that is, to make it disappear. Today, this is certainly possible. Usually the treatment requires injections of gold into your muscles or use of a drug called penicillamine. Some other drugs have been found to induce remission as well. Careful monitoring of all drugs is necessary since side effects are common.

How Are Nonsteroidal Agents Used?

A second group of drugs, nonsteroidal anti-inflammatory agents, are often used to treat RA. These drugs have become very popular for treating RA and other problems as well, including menstrual pain. These drugs affect the chemical mediators that contribute to joint inflammation. In contrast to gold or penicillamine, they work quickly, often bringing relief in hours or days.

One interesting aspect of these drugs is that one may be extremely effective while another may completely fail to bring relief. It may take trial and error to find the drug that is best for you.

Aspirin—Is It Still Effective After All These Years?

If your feet hurt and an arthritic condition is to blame, aspirin is still the benchmark drug to which all other medicines are compared. Today many different and safer forms of aspirin are available.

What About Nondrug Treatment?

Physical therapy, exercise, good nutrition, vitamins, and minerals such as calcium and iron have all been proven to help aching arthritic feet.

Is Surgery Ever an Option?

Surgery ought to be the treatment of last resort. If you haven't responded to other types of treatment for your arthritic feet, occasionally, it can help fuse an unstable ankle joint, for instance. But, fortunately, the vast majority of people will find relief with proper drug therapy, exercise, and vitamin and mineral supplements. Less than 5 percent develop crippling symptoms that require anything as drastic as surgical intervention or, for that matter, a wheelchair.

Chapter 11

Warts

Many of my patients are embarrased to show me the warts on their feet. I remember a 25-year-old model with a beautiful complexion and a successful career who cringed when she took off her shoes because of the warts which covered more than half of the soles of both feet. She had been so mortified about the condition that she had simply hidden her feet for four years while the warts multiplied. And, yes, clusters of warts will continue to grow. But these bumpy, spongy, sometimes thickened, scaly lesions are actually benign little tumors caused by viruses your body hasn't been able to fight off. They are nothing to be embarrassed about, and there are many ways to get rid of them. I admit that there are no simple or 100 percent effective means of ridding yourself of these bothersome lesions, but there is no reason to hide your feet or stumble along in agony. Even the book *Tom Sawyer* has a suggestion, for getting rid of them, "One technique consisted of backing up to the stump, placing the hand with the offending wart into the water, and reciting: 'Barleycorn, barleycorn, Injun-meal shorts; skunk-water, skunk-water, swaller these warts!' "

What Is a Wart?

Warts can appear anywhere on your skin or mucous membranes and can often be painful when they grow on surfaces such as the soles of your feet which are bearing the brunt of your weight. A wart is a benign tumor and is scientifically known as a *verruca*. When it is on the bottom of your foot, we call it a plantar verruca because *plantar* refers to the sole of your foot. In fact, the scientific terms for different warts are simply a way of describing the locations of the warts. For example, warts on your hands are known as verrucae *vulgaris*, differentiating them from the plantar variety on the feet.

Why Are Warts Bothering You?

In my practice, I have found that warts can appear or disappear suddenly, without any effort on your part, or they can survive for years and years. In a study at a state institution for the mentally disabled, untreated warts generally disappeared after about two years, but what often happened was that new warts appeared. However, five years for this hopscotch wart growth seemed to be the limit.

When the wart does give signs of disappearing without any intervention, it may become red, swell, or develop a black, hardened look, or it may simply shrink up. Sometimes when one wart fades away, others nearby will follow suit. They can also proliferate in an uncontrolled way. Warts on different parts of your body often look different, but in each case, a virus called the human papilloma virus, or HPV, is the culprit.

But warts are certainly peculiar. Even though it has been shown that warts can be contagious, I have never had a wart in all my years of treating and touching the warts of my patients. Yet my associate has repeatedly developed single warts on the tips of her fingers even though she carefully cleanses her hands after patient examinations.

Warts often appear on areas of the feet after repeated trauma.

Plantar warts have been known to invade entire schools because children are particularly susceptible to this virus. But the real truth about warts is that there are just no hard truths.

How Do You Know If You Have a Wart?

Some of my patients have been surprised when they first felt what seemed to be a small stone in their shoe near a bony pressure point. It hurt, and they thought it was something they could shake out of their shoe. Many self-diagnosed it as something other than a wart. Sometimes overlying corns or calluses can disguise a plantar wart. A very simple test for a wart is to squeeze the lesion, putting a side-to-side pressure on it. This will hurt. If it were a corn or a callus, the pressure wouldn't be as painful. Another simple test for identifying a wart is to scrape the topmost layer of the lesion. If you see tiny, dark spots resembling dried up blood you are probably looking at capillaries which have been trapped by the wart and have grown in irregular patterns. Warts can bleed profusely because of the presence of these capillaries, so do be careful in your examination.

Are There Different Kinds of Plantar Warts?

Yes, even on the feet, all warts are not the same. There are three basic types. The first is the single, isolated wart, which can range from a tiny dot to a bigger, callused, bothersome blotch 2 to 3 centimeters in diameter. The second variety is the mother-daughter group. The first and larger wart is called the "mother." The warts that appear surrounding this "mother" are sometimes referred to as "daughters." The third type is the mosaic plantar wart, which is a cluster of many warts grouped together on the heel or over the balls of the feet. If you were to examine any of these warty growths under an electron microscope, you could even see the tiny virus particles which thicken the skin and are causing the problem.

Can You Cure Yourself of Warts?

I can think of at least ten ways to attack your warts . . . to which you or your grandmother can probably add a few more. (A friend of mine simply cuts a plain old uncooked potato in half, rubs the wart with the juicy side of the vegetable, and then buries the potato in a sunny spot. Do the warts disappear? Of course. Why? I don't know.)

1. *Salicylic acid pads.* Purchase a packet of 40% to 60% salicylic acid pads at your local drug store. If you can't find them on the shelf, ask. The pharmacist probably has them behind the counter. This is a good wart-remover for young children.

Cut the pad to the size of the wart. Then peel off the paper protecting the sticky side of the pad. Attach the cut pad to your wart and cover it with a bandage to keep it in place and dry. If you manage to repeat this technique six to eight times, your wart won't have much of a chance to survive. Each time you remove the pad to replace it with a new one, you'll notice some deadened tissue. Take a pumice stone or an abrasive brush and scrape this off. Then apply a new piece of acid pad and cover it with another bandage. (*Caution:* The only problem that might occur is if the plaster pad is too large for the wart, and normal, healthy tissue becomes macerated. So do not be careless. Make sure the plaster pad is as close to the size of the wart as possible.)

2. *Compound W.* This is a commercial salicylic acid preparation consisting of acetic acid, menthol, and castor oil. It is a very useful product that is similar to the salicylic-type plaster pad. The medication works best when applied directly to the wart twice a day for up to two weeks. (*Caution:* Be careful to limit its application to the wart; do not apply it to the normal issue.)

3. *Duofilm:* Duofilm is a preparation similar to Compound W but stronger. This commercial salicylic acid preparation is applied directly to the warty material for up to two weeks twice a day until normal tissue reappears. (*Caution:* Apply *only* as directed to avoid damage to surrounding tissue.)

4. *60% Salicylic acid ointment*. This is a good ointment which contains the same substances as other salicylic acid preparations.

5. *Vitamin A*. Injecting vitamin A into the warty material has in some cases dried the wart up.

6. *Phenol*. This is a caustic substance which should only be applied by a doctor since it can cause very painful burns.

7. *Nitric acid, sulfuric acid, and silver nitrate*. Because they are caustic, these should be applied by a doctor.

(Try either Compound W or Duofilm before using these more caustic medications.) Keep your foot as dry as possible if you are using any of treatments 1 through 7. Swimming or bathing will inactivate all the caustic effects of the wart preparations by diluting the concentrations.

8. *Ultrasound*. Ultrasound is nothing more than mechanical waves that are converted into deep heat. It can be administered in a doctor's office for up to three minutes three times per week. It should not be used on growing children, since ultrasound can cause problems when used over the epiphyseal plates (the cartilagenous structure through which the growth of bone occurs). This treatment is best used for adults who do not mind coming in for treatments three times a week.

9. *Surgery*. Surgical excision under local anesthesia works best with the isolated wart when the patient, for one reason or another, wants it out promptly. This procedure may cause scarring due to electrodessication.

10. *Lasers*. This is the newest procedure in the treatment of recalcitrant warts. A laser is simply a device which generates an intense beam of light. The letters in laser stand for *l*ight *a*mplification by *s*timulated *e*mission of *r*adiation. The light emitted in a carbon dioxide laser beam is in the infrared portion of the color spectrum. This means that most living tissues, especially warts, will readily absorb the beam directed at them. The abnormal warty material is killed by the heat of this infrared light.

After local anesthesia numbs the wart, the laser beam is directed around the periphery of the wart. At that point, the warty center can simply be scooped out and any bleeding stopped using an absorbable sterile sponge like Gelfoam.

Chapter 12
Athlete's Foot

Even if you aren't an athlete, you can end up with an athlete's foot, because these funny funguses definitely do not save themselves for the physically fit. In fact, I would say that athlete's foot is one of the least prejudicial diseases I know.

What Exactly Is Athlete's Foot

The technical name for athlete's foot—*tinea pedis*—will probably make a world of difference to your understanding of this peeling, cracking, itching affliction. *Tinea* means "grub, larva, or worm" in Latin and can refer to many different kinds of fungal infections of the skin. *Pedis* lets you know that you are talking about the feet. There are at least four fungal culprits to consider when you think you've got athlete's foot: *Trichophyton rubrum, Trichophyton mentagrophytes, Epidermophyton floccosum,* or *Candida albicans.* But I mention these scientific names only to forewarn you in case a doctor brings them up in your presence. They all mean you've got something we Americans call athlete's foot.

If Athletes Aren't the Only People Who Get This Affliction, Who Else Does and Why?

You are most likely to develop athlete's foot if you are past 65 years of age, overweight, suffering from any kind of circulatory disease, or your usual shoes create a warm, moist, airtight environment for your feet. The organisms which are attacking the skin of your feet and those prime areas between your toes are easily picked up in locker rooms where people have temporarily abandoned their sneakers and socks.

How Do You Know Your Problem Is One of These Funguses?

When I see a patient with a foot condition resembling tinea pedis, I first scrape some of the scaly skin and put it through a laboratory culture test. A solution of potassium hydroxide is combined with the scraping. If one of the funguses is present, the culture will grow. Under a microscope I can tell exactly what is present. Another procedure, using the Wood's light, helps in distinguishing a bacterial infection called erythrasma from athlete's foot. Under this light, the skin scales will fluoresce a coral red if erythrasma is present.

When Is Athlete's Foot a Big Deal, If Ever?

If you assume athlete's foot will go away of its own accord, you can be in big trouble. If a fungal infection goes unchecked, cracks in the skin can develop which allow bacteria to enter, leading to a bacterial infection. One of my patients, a young man in his early twenties, had a fungal infection between his fourth and fifth toes. He tried to ignore it and didn't even keep it dry, powdered, or out of locker rooms. After two weeks, he ended up with a much more severe infection of bacterial cellulitis that put him into the hospital and definitely out of the running.

Why Do Some People Get This All the Time?

These funguses are definitely attracted to some individuals and not others, and your own immune system is to credit or blame. The surface of your skin also makes you more or less susceptible. The more alkaline your skin, as opposed to acidic, the more likely you are to get fungal infections. Another factor may be poor circulation.

Weather can also be a contributing factor. If you live in a warm-all-year-round climate, you are probably more prone as well. These organisms breed best when they've got warmth and moisture to help them along

What Are the Best Treatments?

Keep your feet dry with daily applications of cornstarch or powder. Become fanatical about drying between your toes after your shower or bath. Expose your feet to air and sunlight whenever you can. Don't walk around locker rooms or swimming pool areas barefooted. Change your socks often during each day, and stick with white socks if possible, because colored socks will contribute to heat buildup inside your shoes. The dye in colored socks may also be adding to your fungus problem. Put some powder into your shoes or sneakers before you put them on. Keep one of the following over-the-counter preparations on hand: Tinactin, Halotex, and any of the Desenex products— antifungal ointment, powder, soap, or spray powder. For severe cases, a doctor may prescribe clotrimazole (Lotrimin cream or lotion) or an oral antibiotic such as griseofulvin. However, both of these drugs may cause rash or blistering, and griseofulvin is associated with such side effects as headaches, nausea, and a lessening of sensation in the extremities, so they should be used with care.

Chapter 13
Smelly, Sweaty Feet

Sweat—that salty, clear liquid with your own characteristic odor—is the body's remarkable way of maintaining an even temperature. If it weren't for the act of sweating, your skin would always be colliding environmentally with the hot and cold of the outside world. Like Goldilocks trying to eat the three bears' porridge, you would always be saying, "Too hot" or "Too cold!" But where, when, and how much you sweat is controlled by your nervous system. And sometimes there is an upheaval in this chain of command. Signals get crossed.

What Is This Problem Technically Called?

Bromhidrosis is the term used to describe the excessive secretion of smelly sweat. The word comes from the Greek *bromos*, meaning "stench," and *hidros* meaning "sweat." In relation to your feet it is sometimes called the "dirty sock" syndrome. Bromohidrosis is a quasimedical problem, because it's not serious medically speaking, but it can cause social agony. However, if the sweating problem is severe and blisters develop on your feet as a result of the sogginess, it is called *dyshidrosis,* a more serious, medical condition.

What Causes It?

The exocrine, or sweat, glands found on the soles of your feet and the palms of your hands normally produce perspiration in small amounts. Perspiration is composed of water, sodium chloride, fat, minerals, and various acids that are metabolic end products produced by your body. When bacteria act upon these sweaty secretions, you've got foot odor.

Emotional problems can increase the amount of perspiration. Your body temperature can also trigger an outpouring of sweat; sweating is essential for keeping your body temperature normal. This is the reason why you sweat more when you are exercising.

Closed shoes aggravate sweaty feet and set up a perfect environment for bacteria to grow, leading to more odor and more sweat.

Who Gets Smelly, Sweaty Feet?

Almost all of my patients have at some time or another worried about foot odor. They often apologize to me, "I really did wash my feet today, but they sure do smell."

Disorders in sweating are common in all age groups. Sometimes there is an abnormality in the way the nerves supply the sweat glands with information. Any damage to, or destruction of, nerve endings can cause an increase in perspiration. I've known of severe cases in which an individual produced a full pint of perspiration each week. Normally, the amount is trivial, not even measurable.

Can Food Make Your Feet Smell Funny?

When you eat spicy or pungent foods, such as onions, peppers, garlic, or scallions, the essence of these odors can be excreted through the exocrine glands in your feet. Yes, your feet can end up smelling like what you have eaten.

How Can You Control This Flood and Its Odor?

The key to controlling bromhydrosis is to use either an anti-perspirant or a deodorant right on your feet. Most foot deodorants, like the ones you use under your arms, contain antibacterial agents that can kill the bacteria. They won't stop the perspiring, but they will eliminate the odor. On the other hand, if you choose an antiperspirant, you'll stop the flood and kill the smell at the same time. You might also be interested in trying a menthol antibacterial spray. These have a very cooling effect. Sometimes cornstarch helps, and you can also use your underarm products on your feet.

Here is a list of products designed specifically for the feet. Check the labels before you buy anything, and note that a good odor-prevention product should contain aluminum chloride hexahydrate.

Johnson & Johnson Deodorant Foot Powder contains cornstarch as well as alcohol and antibacterial agents.

Quinsana Deodorant Foot Powder is made of talc, which absorbs perspiration, and tricosan, an antibacterial agent.

Dr. Scholl's Deodorant Spray contains several key ingredients such as zinc phenolsulfonate and a disinfectant that helps some of my patients.

Johnson's Foot Soap contains borax and iodine.

Dr. Scholl's Foot Powder features boric acid.

Dr. Scholl's Deodorant Refresher comes in a spray.

Johnson's Odor-Eaters is a product you may have seen on television because the manufacturer touts its active ingredient as "activated charcoal." This can absorb moisture and has helped some patients.

Other Strategies to Stop the Stench?

Change your shoes and socks as often as you can. Wear light-colored or white all-natural-fiber socks or stockings. Stay away from rubber-soled shoes which don't allow your feet to breathe easily. Wash your feet often and dry them meticulously.

Europeans have been known to sprinkle sage, a leafy herb, into their shoes. Perhaps a dash of these dry, crumbled leaves will do the trick for you.

What If the Sweating Is So Severe That Blistering Has Become Painful?

Sometimes an anticholinergic drug may help. Ask your podiatrist about it. Such a drug blocks the impulses in your nervous system that make you perspire so much. As a last resort, surgery can be performed on your sympathetic nervous system, but this should definitely not be considered until the last. The operation is called a *sympathectomy*.

Chapter 14
The Dry Skin Syndrome

Each cell of your skin in the epidermal or outermost layer is more than 70 percent water. If you were able to wring all the water out of one of these cells, the cell would almost disappear, which is exactly what happens to the cells on the bottoms of your feet as they dry out from the everyday beating they take: they flake away.

Why Does Your Skin Dry Out?

Extreme dryness is really a symptom of an intrinsic change in your skin. It's not a disease all by itself. For instance, in older patients, the rate of new cell growth at the epidermal layer is decreased, and this is partly responsible for the drying. There aren't as many plump new cells forming, and the older cells are losing what water they do have. It should be noted that older cells lose water at a quicker rate than new cells.

Another intrinsic change that comes with older age is decrease in sweating. Your oil glands secrete less and less sebum as you get older, and this contributes to the drying process and to the gradual thinning of the connective tissue in the skin.

Why Are Feet So Vulnerable to Dryness?

Next to your shin bone, your feet, especially your heels, are the most likely victims of the dry skin syndrome. Feet take an incredible amount of pressure, which traumatizes them and may alter their ability to stay soft. Excess callus builds up to protect your feet from the bumps and bruises, and callus is a very dry, tough concentration of skin cells. It doesn't like water.

There are several disorders which may be causing your dry skin problem.

The Dry Skin Disorders

Too Much Keratinization

Sometimes dry skin is due to a process called *keratinization*. Keratin is one of the principal proteins in the cells which make up the surface of your body. It's in your hair, your nails, the enamel of your teeth, and, especially, your skin. In a skin cell, it is not the main ingredient. Because it doesn't easily absorb water, too much keratin can cause problems for your skin even if you moisturize with creams and plain water regularly. The excess keratin keeps water out of the cells; hence you get dry skin. Why excess keratin develops is a biochemical mystery. It may be a congenital disorder. But it's not a hopeless situation. There are products called *keratolytic agents* which contain a small concentration of salicylic acid. These agents will help prevent overkeratinization and force your cells to accept more moisture.

Eczema

Eczema, a word that describes a variety of skin rashes, is an inflammatory disease of the skin. If you've got it, you'll notice lesions, occasional watery discharges from your skin cells, and crusty scabs, and you may be restless, itchy, and running a low-grade fever. Sometimes eczema is caused by an allergy or some other disease you may or may not know you have. For instance, poor leg circulation could cause eczema on your legs and feet, and the poor circulation would tell you that you had a more serious vascular problem that needed to be diagnosed.

Xeroderma

This is the mildest kind of dry skin, and I see it often in older people during the winter months. The lower humidity wreaks havoc on those moisture-starved skin cells, and frequent and meticulous bathing aggravates the problem. Since xeroderma is a condition which disappears when the season changes, the cure is not complicated. I recommend the use of moisturizers on a regular basis to alleviate dryness.

Atopic Dermatitis

This is a condition that shows up in very young people and often in asthma victims. Hay fever and other allergies seem to be associated with this type of dermatitis. If you've got it, red, scaly, itchy patches on your hands and feet will be bothering you. Don't believe that they aren't related to your wheezing. They are. But don't scratch, because chronic aggravation of the patches will make the skin thicker and rougher in those areas.

Athlete's Foot

You may not have considered it, but the fungus between your toes that makes those warm, moist areas so painfully cracked could also be causing the general outbreak of dryness all over.

Psoriasis

The dry rash associated with psoriasis is inherited. You can blame your genes for the red and pink pimples and the white scales they produce. The condition usually strikes the scalp, elbows, knees, arms, legs, and, of course, the feet. It loves the heel area and the soles of your feet, and may even invade the spaces between your toes. Cracks between the toes can make walking very painful.

How Do You Treat Dry Skin?

Since we are really talking about a symptom, let's talk about relieving symptoms here instead of curing diseases. First the general tips: Use a humidifier in your home during winter months. It puts moisture into the air your skin is breathing. Go barefoot more often in your own home. Next, avoid extrahot water in your bath or shower and try using bath oil regularly. Try skipping your bath routine altogether some days. You are losing the water from your surface skin cells by cleaning them too often. Don't buy harsh deodorant soaps anymore, and look for a superfatted brand like Basis or Lubriderm.

External treatments for *psoriasis* include rubbing in 2% to 6% salicylic acid in a petroleum base and applying petroleum jelly to patches; application of tar ointments such as Meditar; and application of steroid preparations to individual plaques. Systemic treatments may consist of methotrexate given by injection once a week or PUVA (photochemotherapy with A-type ultraviolet light). The latter has been in use in some hospitals and special clinics since 1974.

How to Make Your Cream Work Better

I have found that any cream, especially an emollient, which is one that leaves an oil film, will work better when you cover it with plastic wrap overnight. Doris Day, the freckle-faced actress with the skin much younger than her age, used petroleum jelly on a nightly basis. And while she didn't wear a plastic bag to bed, she did cover as much skin as she could with a flannel nightgown. Cortisone cream for a topic dermatitis and antifungal agents for athlete's foot or psoriasis will relieve your symptoms faster if they are covered over while they are absorbed. The only caution about occlusion is for keratolytic agents: salicylic acid under wraps might not be appropriate.

Remember: Take tepid showers and pat your clean skin dry, don't rub it; rough toweling may only dry your skin further. Use emollient soaps and lotions.

Chapter 15
A Cracked Heel

Heel fissures remind me of geological faults. When you let your feet dry till they're parched, they crack. They may not look like San Andreas fault lines, but the deep cracks can make you miserable.

Why Does the Skin at the Back and Bottom of Your Heel Dry Out So Easily and Then Crack?

Your heels need moisture. Callus, which is basically an inelastic, stiff tissue, builds up at the back of your foot where it repeatedly strikes the ground, and this callus needs all the help you can give it to stay soft and under control. If the area becomes too dried out and you keep putting pressure on it, it will crack. The clefts in the callus and the areas of stiff skin on the heel vary in size.

There are other dermatological conditions which will add to your problem, however. Here are just a few:

Psoriasis, as I explained in "The Dry Skin Syndrome," is a chronic skin disease sometimes characterized by scales on your feet as well as changes in your nails. Psoriasis is a primary cause of cracked heels.

Fungal infections can also cause callused, cracking heels.

Hyperkeratosis, or a buildup of callus and dry skin, can produce painful fissures.

Keratoma climacterium is a problem found in short, overweight women who are near menopause.

Overweight, in itself, can cause dry heels as well.

How Do You Treat Cracked Heels?

The first step is to break down the hard, callused skin around the heels, using salicylic acid. This acid, usually in a 60% strength, must be carefully applied and covered with an occlusive dressing. A doctor will do this.

The next step is to use a cream like Whitfield's ointment or cortisone and some plastic wrap for your own occlusive dressing, which will keep moisture from evaporating and increase penetration of the creams. Skin creams should be applied two to three times each day. Hydrisinol and Carmol HC, which contain urea, are excellent moisturing agents. Other good products are Aquacare/HP, Lubriderm, and Eucerin.

When the skin on your heels has softened considerably or has been decallused by the doctor, you should continue to use a pumice stone to abrade any dead skin as it builds up.

How Can You Tell If It Is Psoriasis and Not Athlete's Foot?

If it is a fungus, your toes are likely to be involved, too. Psoriasis, less likely to involve the toes, is characterized by silvery, gray, dry, and patchy lesions.

Will Heel Inserts in Your Shoes Help Stop Cracking?

Sometimes heel inserts help. You might also consider heel cups made of plastic. Sometimes simply eliminating open-backed shoes will cut down on the buildup of callus and subsequently cracking heels.

Chapter 16
More Heel Hurts

In days of yore a pain in the heel was typically attributed to gonorrhea, sore throat, infected sinuses, or a urinary tract infection. And even though thanks to modern medicine, you won't find these associations today, it is still true that when your heel hurts, you hurt all over.

What Is the Most Common Reason for Pain in the Heel?

Most of the time, your heel hurts because you have a heel spur. This is a bony protrusion on the bottom of your foot caused by a growth of calcium that has begun to project downward and is touching your plantar fascia. If you remember, the plantar fascia is that thick piece of tissue underneath the skin on the sole of your foot which extends from your heel to the ball of your foot.

When you begin to feel pain, the plantar fascia is tearing where it is attached to your heel. Because of the pushy protrusion, your arch is being stretched beyond its normal length. There may even be bleeding and further calcification. The calcification can be seen on an x-ray, and what it means is that calcium deposits are building up around the bony point, making it hurt even more. The foot muscles at your heel and along the bottom of your foot are also being strained.

Why Does a Heel Spur Form in the First Place

A heel spur is your body's reaction to stress and strain. Any degree of weight gain, even 10 pounds, if you put it on in a short period of time, can produce greater stress on your arch and lead to the development of a heel spur. Sometimes, a sagging arch adds to the stress. And sometimes shoes with too little room in the arch area are the problem. Any activity which puts excess pressure on your heels—such as jogging, tennis, or paddleball— can cause a heel spur.

Why Does Your Heel Spur Hurt More after You've Been Resting and Not the Reverse?

If you've got a heel spur, you've probably noticed how contrary it is immediately after you wake up in the morning and set your foot on the floor. Heel spur pain is always greatest after rest and will improve after you walk for a few minutes. This is because you are straining your plantar fascia when you put your foot on the floor. It had been at rest while you slept, and when the heel spur stresses it anew, it registers pain. If your heel spur is inflamed because of a fluid-filled bursal sac next to the bone, it may make your whole leg ache.

What Can You Do to Ease the Pain?

If your pain is acute, take an analgesic like Tylenol or another over-the-counter pain killer. Rest is also important because it will help reduce the inflammation around the spur. Elevating your foot and applying ice to the heel for twenty minutes at a time are also helpful. The next thing I usually recommend is a foam or felt heel pad cut in a U shape to match your heel shape. When your immediate pain has subsided, losing weight, getting a special orthotic made to fit your heel, and learning how to keep your heel cushioned inside your shoe are often in order.

What If Nothing Seems to Help?

If my conservative recommendations don't work, go to the podiatrist, who can offer you ultrasound pain therapy, electrogalvanic stimulation, or special footbaths. If these techniques don't work, you may need surgery. Heel spur surgery is designed to correct whatever biomechanical problem is causing the spur in the first place. For this reason, it would be difficult for me to tell you exactly what a surgeon might do. Each case differs slightly from the next. Sometimes a surgeon simply shaves off or removes the excess calcium deposit.

MRS. B'S BRUISE

Normally, Mrs. B walked ten blocks to and from her job each day wearing her sneakers. One day, however, she developed a sharp, shooting pain on the bottom of her foot which felt like a "bruise." This very bruised sensation sent pain right up into her arch from her heel, where it was the worst. She came into my office on crutches.

As I carefully reviewed her medical history, the fact that she had recently gained an extra 15 pounds came out. A vacation had sent the scales climbing. When I x-rayed her foot, I saw a large heel spur on her right foot.

What to do? I injected a local anesthetic plus Celestone (betamethasone), which is an anti-inflammatory drug, directly into her heel. To help her avoid pressure on the soft tissue around the little spur, I gave her what is called an immobilization strap that would raise her heel ¼ inch up with its padding. She started to take Tylenol right away and regularly. On her second visit a few days later, I designed an orthotic shoe insert of soft, compressible material cut to the shape of her heel, and I told her to stop wearing her sneakers for the time being. The sneakers hadn't been offering her heel enough arch support. Whenever she went shoe shopping thereafter, she looked for good arch support, and now, six months later, still wearing her orthotics, she is pain free.

Is There Anything Else That Can Cause Heel Pain?

Yes, sometimes there is an abnormal clump of tissue at the back of your heel, just over the bone, called a Haglund deformity. This is the proverbial "pump bump," and I see it in two types of feet: the very high arched foot and the very low arched foot. What happens is that the back of the shoe is continually rubbing against the bump, irritating the area. One of those inflamed, fluid-filled bursal sacs may result.

By applying warm heat—a wet face towel, for instance—or a heating pad to the spot, you can ease the situation. Do this several times a day, and be careful when you buy shoes. Some sufferers also use heel pads. By placing heel pads in your shoes to lift your foot almost out of the shoe, you can avoid the irritation. Shoes with soft edges are a good idea, too. The hardened edge of an ordinary shoe can be murder for someone with a Haglund deformity.

On rare occasions, a hurting heel can be the result of pressure on one of your nerves, the *tarsal tunnel syndrome*. If a podiatrist can't find a heel spur, this is a diagnosis to be considered. The nerve involved passes through your ankle near a ligament which leads to your heal. When something is pressuring it—perhaps because of a biomechanical shift—it will send pain right down to your heel.

Chapter 17
Allergies

They may not be able to sniffle, sneeze, or wheeze, but your feet, just like any other part of your body, can be affected by allergies.

What Does a Foot Allergy Look Like?

Your feet usually react to an offending allergen with an instant case of *contact dermatitis*. Those red, bumpy, swollen spots are ugly and they hurt. *Contact* is the key word in this definition, of course, and the edges of your outbreak will be clear-cut. Does your rash stop at the same spot your shoes end? Or can you clearly see the outline of your offending socks after you've removed them?

Why Has It Happened?

Did you recently purchase a new pair of shoes, stockings, socks? If you are allergic to nickel for instance, you will also react to substances called chromates, used in the shoe-dying and leather-curing process. Or, you may be allergic to the main ingredient in rubber cement, mercaptobenzothiazole, which is used to put pieces of leather together in a shoe. Various leather dyes also treat feet poorly and can bring on an eruption of blisters and bumps.

Can You Have an Allergic Reaction That Starts Slowly and Builds Up to a Painful Pitch All Over the Skin Surface?

Yes. You can have an allergic rash all over after wearing a new pair of shoes or socks and walking or sitting in a warm environment for a while. Friction and heat can combine with allergies to create a veritable war zone.

Moisturizing creams containing neomycin, lanolin, penicillin, perfumes, preservatives (e.g., sulfates), antihistamines, and paragens may all be anathema. Read ingredient labels and stay away from these substances if your feet break out after applying them once.

How Can You Find the Awful Allergen?

If guesswork hasn't given you a clue, go for a patch test at the doctor's office. This may pinpoint the offending chemical. One of my patients, a twenty-six-year-old woman with dry, cracking heels, had applied a lanolin cream to her heels to soothe the dryness. Little did she realize what a reaction she was about to set off. The lanolin, to which she was allergic, wreaked havoc on her feet.

How Bad Can a Foot Allergy Be?

Pretty bad. When a twenty-seven-year-old chef came to see me, still wearing his rubber-soled shoes, my heart went out to him. Red, swollen, oozing feet indicated the most severe case of contact dermatitis I had ever seen. What he didn't realize was that his comfortable work shoes with the rippled soles were the reason his feet were on fire.

How Do You Get Rid of the Painful Reaction?

If the allergy won't subside easily, you may want to see an allergist. Often a corticosteroid medication is in order. Steroids are widely used drugs which are often prescribed in injectable doses. They are produced by your own adrenal glands but can be manufactured synthetically in a laboratory. Steroids reduce inflammation and can be a big help in controlling allergic or rheumatic reactions. Steroids, however, can also affect your metabolism negatively, so you should be careful. Patients on steroids for long periods of time run the risk of raising their blood sugar levels, retaining high amounts of salt, lowering their body's resistance to infection, and other serious complications. A steroid prescribed for contact dermatitis, though, is less potentially dangerous, because it is used topically, not injected.

Once the rash subsides, footbaths can be very soothing.

THE FOOT TEATIME TRICK

Place your feet in a bathtub or pail of warm water (100° F or 38° C) with three tea bags. Tea is an excellent source of soothing tannic acid. Soak your feet for at least twenty minutes. If you take this tea break at least three times a week, you can eliminate part of your foot perspiration problem, which undoubtedly contributes to your allergic response.

Can You Be Allergic to All Shoes?

The first thing you've got to do is control perspiration. The tea trick, dusting with cornstarch, and other moisture-control measures are a must. If your rashes are really bad and you can't find shoes, write to the Alden Shoe Company, Tauton Street,

Middleborough, Massachusetts 02346. They specialize in shoes that are made without chromates and use no rubber cement.

HOW BLOOD FLOW AFFECTS YOUR FEET

Because circulation of blood down to the very tips of your toes is so very important for keeping you healthy, I decided to turn to a vascular specialist for a more complete explanation of circulation and the feet. Dr. Harry Schanzer is Professor of Surgery at Mount Sinai School of Medicine, New York City, and director of the vascular laboratory there.

Blood performs many services for the legs and feet: It brings oxygen and nutrients to the tissues and takes away wastes. The arteries, capillaries, and veins provide a route for the blood. When disease causes the arteries and veins to narrow, all sorts of problems can arise, ranging from mild pain to life-threatening clots and aneurysms. Here are a few problems you should be aware of, according to Dr. Schanzer:

Arterial Problems

Acute Ischemia.   When a sudden blockage of an artery slows blood flow so that cells can no longer function, acute ischemia may occur. You will feel sudden pain in the leg or foot, and your lower leg will look pale and feel cold. You won't be able to feel a pulse. You must have immediate treatment to open the clogged artery. Your physician will do this by removing the clot (thrombectomy) or doing a bypass around the narrowed area.

Chronic Ischemia   Artery blockage can be so slight that pain or leg cramps will appear only during exercise, after you walk for a while, for instance. The more severe the problem, the shorter the distance you'll be able to walk. Exercise and stopping smoking help in mild cases.

Some people have pain even while resting, or have ulcerations or gangrene. They are in danger of losing the leg and foot, and must undergo aggressive treatment. An x-ray of the arteries (an arteriogram) will reveal the blood's "roads and blocks" and will indicate the best way to treat the blockage. In one procedure, a catheter with a balloon tip is placed into the artery (no surgery is needed for this), and the balloon is inflated, pushing open the artery. In more severe cases, bypass surgery or surgical division of the sympathetic nerves can be used.

Vein (Venous) Problems

Veins contain valves that help the blood return to the heart. Blood clots within the veins (thrombophlebitis) and malfunctions of the valves are the two greatest problems found in the veins.

Thrombophlebitis   Small clots can form in small veins close to the skin (superficial thrombophlebitis) or deep in the large veins of the leg (deep venous thrombosis).

If you have varicose veins, you may be subject to superficial thrombophlebitis, which is characterized by painful, localized, red, hot, and swollen veins, due to small clots. Sometimes you can even feel a tender lump. Your best bet is to place heat on the swollen vein, and take aspirin for the pain. Within ten to fifteen days, all symptoms should be gone.

Deep-vein thrombosis is serious. Not only does the clot cause pain and a great deal of swelling, it can also break off and travel through the veins to the lungs, producing an embolism. This can be fatal. Thus, diagnosis and treatment are very important, and require help from an experienced vascular specialist. These emboli are treated with bed rest and anticoagulant drugs such as heparin and Coumadin.

Another serious problem that can occur is "venous gangrene." Without proper treatment, the lower leg and foot may have to be amputated.

Spider and Varicose Veins.   These trouble many women, particularly, and are caused by valve malfunctions. (Remember, the valves are essential for blood to return to the heart.) When the valves don't work just right, blood will not circulate properly and the veins can become swollen and twisted. This is what causes a varicose vein. For most persons, this is only a cosmetic problem, and there are no symptoms. If the veins are small and cause no problems, nothing needs to be done. If you are bothered by the way they look, however, you can have sclerosant injections into the veins. These injections cause a chemical inflammation, making the walls of the veins stick together. After the inflammation has vanished, the varicose veins will not be noticeable. If they are very large, however, they can be surgically treated. In either case, remember that these veins can come back again.

In a few cases, varicose veins can produce much discomfort, can cause superficial phlebitis, and can bleed profusely if ruptured.

Spider veins, or superficially dilated capillaries, are almost always seen only in women. They are harmless, and if they are abundant, small, and affect a large area of the legs and feet, they can be hidden with makeup. If they occur in one area and are connected to a vein, they can be injected in the same way as varicose veins. However, this takes many sessions, and demands a great deal of patience on your part and your doctor's part as well.

Chronic Venous Stasis   When valves in important veins in the leg or foot break down, swelling, dark pigmentation, and painless leg ulcers can appear. The best way to treat this is with custom-fitted pressure-gradient elastic stockings or special surgery to correct the defect in the valve.

Lymphatic Disease   Lymphatics are small vessels that remove water and excess proteins from the tissues. As they move up the foot and leg, they find "resting stations," or lymph glands, and finally drain into the veins. If they are blocked or missing, fluids rich in proteins will pool in the tissues, causing a swollen, hard, thick-skinned leg and foot. This is called *lymphedema*, and in its most terrible form is called elephantiasis. Some of the causes of blocked lymph flow include surgery or radiation therapy.

Chapter 18

Burning Soles

After seven blocks of city walking in new sandals last summer, I felt like one of the firewalkers—that new breed of third-degree sensation seekers—because the bottoms of my feet were on fire.

What Makes the Bottoms of Your Feet Feel Hot, Itchy, and Painful?

A constant burning sensation on both soles is clearly due to a serious disease with its origin somewhere other than your feet, but the key word here is *constant*, meaning both day and night. I sometimes see patients with a burning sensation that is similar but has been caused by wearing certain shoes—like the sandals that put me in agony last summer. Non-porous, probably man-made, inner soles are usually to blame. Leather, suede, or plain old cotton canvas don't often cause this sort of problem. Bare feet are especially vulnerable; alternatively, the burn may result from an incorrect fit; friction inside a shoe that doesn't allow your foot to breathe easily can cause the pain.

Really constant burning, however, indicates that you have injured the nerve endings on the bottoms of both feet. Drugs and chemicals can be responsible. I recall one patient who developed this burning, itching sensation the day after he had been treated with a drug called heparin for another disorder. Ingestion of arsenic, mercury, lead, or any of the so-called heavy metals can also mimic a viral infection that will reach your feet in the long run.

What Kind of Diseases Destroy the Nerves in Your Feet?

Alcoholism, pernicious anemia, and diabetes are just three of the more serious diseases that can affect your feet. Alcoholism, in particular, will cause a loss of vitamin B and thiamine in your body and will subsequently damage the nerves of your feet.

If pernicious anemia is causing your problem, I would be able to tell by using a simple tuning fork on a bony point on your foot. I would be looking for your nerve reaction to the feel of the fork. A person suffering from pernicious anemia wouldn't feel anything. Pernicious anemia, which I usually see in older individuals, is more than a low blood count. It involves an intrinsic change in your blood, and produces neurological changes in many parts of your body, not just the soles of your feet. The burning sensation is undoubtedly just one in a cluster of symptoms. To be certain of my diagnosis, however, I'd also order blood tests.

Anyone with lifelong diabetes is inevitably going to face foot problems. The nerve damage this nasty disease brings about is quite insidious, but the first sign of it in your feet is this burning sensation.

How Can You Stop the Pain?

If you know the fault lies with your new shoes, you can either get rid of the shoes or ask a shoe-repair shop to permanently insert a new strip of leather or another all-natural lining. Sometimes this helps and sometimes nothing will, short of a different pair of shoes.

If alcohol is to blame, you can eliminate it and start taking therapeutic doses of vitamin B complex. But check with a doctor first.

If you can't find the root of your problem in anything obvious, and you wonder if you may have come into close contact with a heavy metal, certain blood tests, an analysis of your urine, and a thorough physical examination by a doctor are in order.

Could the Burning Sensation Be Due to the Way You Walk?

Perhaps. If your feet only burn after walking long distances and they seem to burn no matter which shoes you wear, and you've ruled out other more serious medical problems, you're probably correct in guessing some kind of biomechanical problem. Ask a podiatrist or physical therapist to analyze your gait.

Why Do Your Feet Only Burn in the Summer?

The heat, moisture from perspiration, the type of airless shoe you are choosing, and nylon or unnatural fiber socks or stockings are all contributing factors. Go back to square one and start eliminating problems one at a time. One of the laws of physics is that friction equals heat, which, of course, will then create a burning sensation. In the summer, the heat will always be greater than at other times of year.

One way to cut down on this problem is to wear white or light-colored cotton socks in the summer.

Are Burning Feet Found in Older People More Often?

Yes. The older you get, the thinner the fat pads on the bottom of your feet become. Fat is important in controlling friction, so the less fat you have, the hotter *your* feet get from the friction.

Chapter 19
Cold Feet

When was the last time someone told you she had "cold feet" about doing something—getting married, going skiing, having a baby? "Having cold feet" means having a case of nervous jitters. And nerves are one of the keys to the problem of icy cold feet.

Why Are Your Feet Always So Cold?

Your feet get cold because your warm blood isn't circulating properly through the veins and arteries into your legs and out to your toes. Normally, the skin temperature down there should range between 75 and 90°F. If it drops below 65°F, you've got a problem with your vascular, or circulatory, system. Your arteries, the smaller-sized blood vessels called arterioles, and your veins aren't letting enough blood through.

Your nervous system plays a significant part in determining how much blood gets through. If you are disturbed about something or under a great deal of stress, nerves can constrict the little arterioles in your feet and lessen their ability to carry blood, giving you cold feet. At the other emotional extreme is the person ("hot under the collar") whose nervous system sends excess blood through when the pressure is on. This is called vasodilation of the blood vessels, and it can make you hot all over.

How Can Cigarettes Make Your Feet Cold?

Believe it or not, smoking tobacco is a major cause of cold feet. You probably already know that you put your heart and your lungs at risk when you smoke, but you may never have blamed cigarettes for your cold feet. The nicotine makes your blood vessels tighten up, or constrict, and since it works on your entire nervous system, it affects these arterioles in your feet as well as in other areas. When they handed the cigarette and cup of hot coffee to recovering victims in those old movies, they weren't doing them any favors. The warmth of the gesture was the only real warmth extended, because nicotine and caffeine are blood vessel constrictors. Amphetamines, diet pills like Dexatrim, and some other medications work the same way. Take a look at what you are taking in on a regular basis if you want to get clues to your coldness.

Sometimes the local anesthetic you receive in the dentist's chair contains epinephrine, which constricts blood flow, and some over-the-counter allergy remedies for nasal congestion or sniffles include ephedrine, which also contributes to a constricted blood flow and cold feet.

How Bad Can the Blood Flow Really Be?

After inhaling one cigarette, the blood flow to your feet may be reduced by as much as 50 percent! When does it pick up again? Sometimes not for an hour after that single cigarette. So you can imagine what happens if you're smoking two or three packs a day. The more you smoke, the colder you get. What's diabolical about this is that you probably pick up another cigarette to try to warm yourself up.

What Are Some of the Circulatory Disorders
Keeping Your Feet Cold?

Raynaud's Disease: This is a relatively common disorder I see in women between ages twenty and forty whose hands and feet get very cold and even numb on occasion. Toes and fingertips suffer the most. If you have this problem, you undoubtedly already know that the attacks seem to come and go without warning, and winter is your worst time of year. Rest assured. You don't have a serious circulatory disease if your problem has been diagnosed as Raynaud's disease. You simply have an uncomfortable condition that seems to be triggered by cold weather and a bad habit like smoking. Do go to the doctor's office for a professional opinion because your symptoms can mirror those of something more serious with the same first name. *Raynaud's Syndrome* is another matter and something to worry about.

A diagnosis of Raynaud's disease, as I said, should not be cause for too much concern. Simply wearing warm socks and other warm clothes in severely cold weather will keep the situation under control. Avoid open-toed sandals and don't smoke. Look at cigarettes as allergens and stay away from them.

Raynaud's Syndrome: This is a disorder which arises from the inability of your arteries to dilate and send blood where it is supposed to go. The attacks are episodic and seem to be brought on by cold temperatures, much like that of Raynaud's disease. It is linked to various underlying systemic diseases, such as collagen diseases, lead or nicotine toxicity, or neurovascular trauma.

The key to treatment for Raynaud's Syndrome is to avoid the cold. In severe cases, in which the numbing gets out of hand, a physician may suggest a sympathectomy, a surgical procedure in which some sympathetic nerves to the foot or hand are cut. This should only be a last resort, however.

Buerger's Disease: Also known as *thromboangiitis obliterans,* this syndrome shows up in adult men who haven't passed their fortieth birthday. What happens is that the small arteries and arterioles in the legs and feet constrict and refuse to let the proper amount of blood pass through. It is directly related to smoking and the difference between Buerger's and Raynaud's is that with Buerger's disease actual tissue will be destroyed in the long run, turning ulcerous and eventually becoming gangrenous as the disease runs its course.

The fundamental treatment for Buerger's disease is to stay away from smoke of any kind. Don't smoke yourself, and don't inhale the smoke from anyone else's cigarettes if you can help it. Sometimes medication to make your blood vessels open up or dilate is prescribed, but this isn't always very successful. If you have any signs of Buerger's, get rid of the cigarettes; it won't cure the disease, but it will certainly reduce the severe muscle cramps and nocturnal pain associated with the disease.

Will Exercise Help Your Cold Toes?

Yes. Exercise can definitely improve your circulation and warm your feet up. Get out there and start walking. Turn to "Observe Your Lifestyle" in Part Three for more detailed information about exercise.

Is There Any Other Basic Advice for Avoiding Cold Feet?

Never wear constricting undergarments. Stockings that are too tight, underpants which cut painfully into the top of your legs. Girdles don't help your problem at all. Try not to cross your legs when you are sitting down.

Chapter 20
Aching Arches

Generations of specialists were told that good feet could be judged by their arches. A foot with no arch at all—the proverbial flatfoot—was considered poor indeed. But the height of your arches just doesn't carry that kind of weight anymore. Low, high, or middling, your arch is only as excellent as its ability to pronate. And pronation is probably the key to your pain when your arches are aching.

What Does Pronation Mean?

Normally your foot strikes the ground heel first, rolling forward toward your toes and inward at the arch. But your arch should only be dipping a little in this process. If it dips down too much, you've got what podiatrists call excess *pronation*. Your foot should spring back from each step without letting the whole arch touch the ground in a collapsing effect. If your arch falls on you, you're going to have pain.

Why Isn't Your Arch Working Properly?

Sometimes ligaments are to blame, sometimes degenerative arthritic changes in the bones are the cause, and sometimes inherited flat-footedness is your problem. Simply having "flat" feet won't take the spring out of your step but troublesome muscle, bone, and ligament alignment, in which nothing fits together quite right, can make the arch of your foot take the brunt of your weight when you walk. That inner side of your sole wasn't designed to bear the complete burden.

Are There Any Other Reasons for Aching Arches?

If you haven't used your feet much and you suddenly find yourself in a *change of routine* which demands a lot more walking, standing, or climbing of steps, you can also end up with aching arches. In this situation, you've simply overstretched underused muscles. Being unprepared for basketball, jogging, and tennis games have been found to be arch enemies too.

One of the most common causes of arch pain is *plantar fasciitis*, which simply means you have overstretched a band of tissue, called the plantar fascia, running along the bottom of your foot from your heel to the ball of the foot. This band can become inflamed and will be very painful upon walking. Standing on the rung of a ladder or step stool too long is a typical way to hurt your plantar fascia.

Tendinitis, or an inflammation of the small tendons which attach the muscles in your feet to their bones, may also be the cause of your arch pain. Long distance runners have the worst tendon problems I've seen in my practice.

How Do You Treat Arch Pain?

Whether you've got tendinitis, plantar fasciitis, or simply aching arches, the best medicine is *rest first;* then ice packs and, later, heat may be applied to your foot. This should quickly reduce any inflammation. An elastic bandage wrapping may help support the area, and a new pair of shoes with extra arch supports or an orthotic insert can also ease your agony. A wedge raising the inner border of your foot by ⅛ to ¼ inch may be the best solution in the long run, but you are going to want professional advice for this problem.

In fact, if you are still in pain after trying home remedies, a visit to a doctor's office is in order. In certain cases, bones have been known to shift dangerously, and if this is the case, you ought to know about it.

How Can a Doctor Tell Something Is Wrong with Your Arch and the Way You Walk?

A good podiatrist or orthopedist will examine you by asking you to walk and watching your foot fall and your gait as you do so. Then he or she will ascertain your foot's range of motion by rotating it at the ankle and checking it for other kinds of flexible motion. If the doctor doesn't do this but simply relies on your description of symptoms, it's a poor job.

How Long Do You Have to Keep the Pressure Off Your Arches If They Hurt When You Jog?

Stay away from your regular running schedule for at least a week to see if the pain goes away. If it persists, then a visit to the doctor is a must.

THE INFAMOUS FLAT FOOT

There are entire generations of people who were forced to be embarrassed by their flat feet. A foot with no arch was considered inferior . . . possibly even dangerous. Rigid devices were once implanted into the shoes of flat-footed persons. Having flat feet dismissed you from the army. And at the other end of this extremist thinking was the acceptance of the high arch as highly desirable.

All this has changed in recent years. A flat foot, when there is no exaggerated pronation or caving-in of the arches, is actually a fine foot. And, in a reverse trend, an extremely high arch is seen as capable of causing myriad biomechanical problems.

Your arch, for better or for worse, is evaluated on the basis of the way it pronates. Normally your foot strikes the ground from the outside back of your heel first and rolls toward the ball or metatarsal area. As it does, your entire heel should come to rest on the ground as well. Your arch lowers a little in this process. If your foot doesn't work well, the arch falls flat on the ground with a thump. This is what a podiatrist calls being abnormally, and unhealthily, flat. Your arch is not bearing up under your weight. Just because your arch is exceptionally high or low doesn't mean you will have any trouble walking correctly. It's the degree of pronation, or flattening out, that can put you in a podiatrist's red flag category.

Sometimes a knock-kneed individual will have pronated feet. The person's feet are trying to compensate for the shape of such lower legs. Loose ligaments, weak muscles, trouble with an Achilles tendon, and certain other disorders too rare to be worth mentioning here can also make your feet unnaturally flat. You may also inherit inferior flat feet.

But remember, all flat feet are not inferior. They may even be far superior to higher-arched feet because they can absorb the shock of walking over a bigger foot surface.

Chapter 21
Battered Ligaments

Lowly ligaments are always taken for granted. These tough, fibrous tissues which connect bones to each other stand up under extremes of motion without any attention, let alone pampering. You don't even see body builders praising each other for the ligamentous perfection they may have achieved. It's not until you strain or overstretch one that you realize they are just as important as muscle and bone.

What Does a Battered Ligament Feel Like?

By battered, I mean strained, stretched, or impaired in some way. When these fibrous connecting bands are injured, it can be difficult to walk without pain or to move an area without feeling as though something has become disconnected or disjointed. Your ankle is especially prone to such problems. At this joint, which bears the brunt of much of your weight, three bones come together—the talus, the tibia, and the fibula. You can thank two groups of ligaments for the unusual and complete stability of this joint. These groups, called the medial and the lateral ligaments, allow your foot to move up and down. You can't walk without them.

High heels can wreak havoc with these ligaments. In a high-heeled shoe, your plantar flexion, or your ability to flex your foot up and down, is impaired, and the higher the heel, the more vulnerable you are to injury.

What Are the Most Common Types of Ankle Ligament Injury?

When you twist your ankle awkwardly inward and back toward your body, you can strain your lateral ligaments (the group on the outside of your foot). Sometimes this sudden twisting can hurt the medial, or inside, group as well.

Is There a Difference between a Strain and a Sprain?

A *strain* is caused by overstretching a muscle, tendon, or ligament, without any significant tearing. It is considered to be a minor injury with a quick recovery. A *sprain* is a disruption of the joint where there is an actual tearing of ligaments from their attachment points.

Who Is Most Susceptible to Sprains?

You are more likely to sprain your ankle if you are "double-jointed" (if you have been born with excess motion in your joints); if you are overweight; if you are pregnant; or if you play fast sports like tennis or racketball that involve stressful side stretches at the ankle.

How Does Your Extra Weight Relate to Your Ligaments?

If you are overweight, you put increased stress on your weight-bearing joints, especially your ankles. Knees and hips are also problem spots prone to ligamentous injuries.

What Does "Center of Gravity" Have to Do with Your Ligaments?

Try to imagine an invisible line extending up through the middle of your body, past your belly button, and out through the very center of the top of your head. This is often called the line of your center of gravity, and for complete stability, it should be straight. If you've got a permanently slouched shape, if you hang the top of your body to one side or the other, or if you are pregnant, your center of gravity is thrown off. You are stressing those ligaments which support your bones and general shape. You are out of alignment, in other words, and your ligaments are struggling to compensate for this misshaping. They take a beating when this happens, and if you push them too far, you sprain them.

Pregnancy puts extra stress on ligaments because there are two factors working against them: the excess weight all in one spot and the increased amounts of female hormones in your body. These hormones create ligamentous laxity in your body. Ligaments need to relax so you'll have room to accommodate your growing baby and get through labor and delivery, but at the same time the ligaments across your stomach are stretching appropriately, other ligaments are weakened. You may find yourself twisting an ankle or being able to flip your wrist in a way you never could before. Rest assured, it's not a permanent condition.

How Do You Know If You Have a Seriously Sprained Ligament?

If you can't walk after a few minutes of rest, if you can't resume normal activities without any pain, or if you hear a distinct "pop" when you hurt yourself, you know you have torn tissue. Prolonged pain, swelling, a bruised look with its black-and-blueness all mean you should have an x-ray taken.

What If You Can't Get to a Doctor Immediately?

Put ice on the injured area. Keep your leg or foot elevated, and try using an elastic bandage to compress the swelling. The ice will help constrict the blood flow and stop the injury from swelling too much. Raising the area above the level of your heart will enlist the help of gravity in keeping blood away.

What Does a Doctor Ordinarily Recommend?

After I order an x-ray of the area, I usually recommend ice for the first twenty-four to forty-eight hours and an elastic bandage. After several days of this, my patients are advised to soak their ankles in warm water (96 to 100°F) for twenty minutes before beginning simple stretching exercises. Any such stretching is aimed at increasing the range of motion.

How Long Will It Be Before Your Ankle Is Better?

It may take six to eight weeks for a simple sprain to heal. I have treated cases which were severe enough to require a cast and up to twelve weeks of immobilizaton.

Are There Tricks to Avoiding Ligament Sprains?

Yes. If you are exercising or running, wear good footgear. Poorly constructed shoes can do terrible things to your ankles and feet. If you can't get shoes to fit right and feel comfortable, opt for some specially made orthotic inserts.

Don't run on uneven ground, and if you have inherently weak joints or other ligament problems, be careful when you run, jog, breakdance, or play racket sports.

Chapter 22
Achilles Tendinitis

The Achilles tendon, named for Achilles, the Greek hero who was only vulnerable at the back of his heel, is the large tendon at the back of your lower leg attached to the heel. It is actually three individual tendons serving two muscles in your leg.

What Do You Mean by Tendinitis?

Inflammation of a tendon is called tendinitis. But to understand tendinitis better, you need to know how tendons function. All tendons are elastic bands of tissue that attach muscle to bone. When a muscle contracts, the tendon makes the bone move, too. Even though tendons are held in place by connective tissue, there is some latitude for slipping. A good example of this is the popping sound you hear when you crack your knuckles.

The tendons are covered by a smooth tendon sheath, which allows the gliding motion over bone. Since tendons have a poor blood supply, they heal very slowly when they are injured.

How Do You Get Achilles Tendinitis?

This condition is usually caused by some kind of tremendous force being placed upon an inflexible lower leg. For this reason, I see dancers, runners, novice marathoners, and others who try to push themselves too far too fast. Dancers almost always rupture their Achilles tendon just above the site where the muscle attaches to the tendon, or just below the calf.

Others who are prone to this injury are women who wear high heels all the time and suddenly switch to flat shoes. In this case, the muscles in the back of the lower legs have been shortened from wearing high heels too much, and great force is put on the tendons when flats are worn. Simply keeping your lower leg muscles properly stretched can prevent this.

How Do You Know If You Have Achilles Tendinitis?

Pain is the number one symptom. There may be a slight swelling and the base of your heel may be painful to touch. The tissue around the Achilles tendon where it inserts into the heel may appear reddish, and you may also hear the sound of two surfaces rubbing against each other when you move your ankle.

As in ligamentous injuries, there are varying degrees of damage. If you feel sharp pain in your calf, you may have a defect somewhere above your ankle area. If the tendon is mildly hurt, a first-degree case, you will find it difficult to rise up on your toes or walk on your heels. A second-degree case involves partial tearing of the tendon away from the heel bone. In a third-degree injury, the tendon is completely torn away from the bone, and some muscles may be ruptured as well. Only surgery will correct the situation. In the second- and third-degree cases, the ability to ambulate is significantly impaired.

What Can You Do?

Rest your leg. Apply ice to keep the swelling down. Your heel can also be elevated with an insert of felt or foam to eliminate stress on the back of the leg.

What Can the Doctor Do?

Initial treatment for all three degrees of injury includes the use of ice, compression, and elevation for the first twenty-four to forty-eight hours, until a diagnosis can be made. Complete immobilization and sometimes surgery are required. The foot may have to be immobilized for up to eight weeks.

Your doctor will apply heel lifts and will strap your foot with the toes pointed downward and the heel off the ground. When there is a lot of swelling of the tendon sheath, an injection of a steroid, given judiciously, can be helpful. The use of steroids is somewhat controversial, but sometimes they can help, particularly if there is a chance the tendo Achilles will be scarred. Your physician also may place your foot in a flexible cast (such as an Unna boot), to eliminate some of the swelling and to reduce movement around the Achilles tendon insertion.

With a first-degree injury, you will be able to walk after about forty-eight hours, and will have little pain. However, running, dancing, or any kind of strenuous exercise will be virtually impossible for some time. A second-degree injury takes anywhere from six to eight weeks to heal, and an additional three to four weeks for stretching exercises to have an effect before normal activity can resume.

What If Your Pain Persists?

If pain persists after the initial treatments, anti-inflammatory drugs such as aspirin, indomethacin (Indocin), or phenylbutazone (Butazolidin) are recommended.

Can You Avoid This Injury?

The best way to avoid Achilles tendinitis is to keep your body limber and to use general warm-up exercises to stretch the Achilles tendons as well as other parts of the body. A regular stretching program will increase the flexibility of muscles, ligaments, and tendons, and inevitably helps prevent injury.

Chapter 23
Shin Splints

My experience with shin splints is personal as well as professional. After years of a somewhat sedentary life, I started a jogging program, and a doctor who didn't follow her own good advice ended up doctoring herself.

What Exactly Is a Shin Splint?

When you have a shin splint, the two muscles attached to your shin, the front of your lower leg, are pulling away from the bone. Your leg feels tight, perhaps swollen, and hurts when you walk. The connective tissue covering that bone becomes inflamed, and you may have other spots of inflammation on your lower leg.

What Makes the Muscles Pull Away?

If your feet are excessively pronated, the lower leg muscles must work harder to compensate for your inflexible foot. Such an unsound foot makes the muscles strain to keep the foot straight as you jog or run across a tennis court. Sometimes those muscles begin to pull away from the bone. That's when you get a shin splint.

Running on extrahard surfaces, even when you have good foot balance, can put the same kind of pressure on these muscles. Or, if your heel cords are too tight for a new exercise program, you can also send the strain up your leg. Simply lifting your leg off the ground will put tremendous pressure on these particular muscles when all is not quite right anywhere from your feet on up.

Can You Actually Develop a Small Lump from a Shin Splint?

Yes. If your condition is allowed to worsen, the soft tissue on your shin bone can become inflamed. That's what the lump is all about.

Who Gets Shin Splints?

Anyone like me who is a novice sports enthusiast, who hasn't been building up slowly to an exercise regime, or who overdoes it can end up with shin splints. Abnormal stress on these muscles will tighten them and make them pull away from the bone.

How Do You Treat Shin Splints?

The first step is to use ice packs on the inflammed muscles. What you are trying to do is to reduce the inflammation. Then, rest. Finally, before any vigorous activity, it is a good idea to stretch the muscles by flexing your feet slowly up and down. This will certainly reduce the likelihood of shin splints in the future. It may also be helpful to wrap your leg in an elastic bandage to absorb some of the shock you get each time your heel hits the ground; what you want to do is immobilize the joints and bones in your feet. Last, if you are in the midst of a painful bout, try an analgesic.

Are There Any Other Kinds of Pain Associated with the Lower Leg?

Sometimes it's not a shin splint at all but a stress fracture of the lower leg. If your shin splint pain doesn't go away with ice, rest, and easy stretching, go to a doctor for an x-ray. That's the only way to detect a fracture. Stress fractures don't always call for a cast, but they always need to be diagnosed and treated by a doctor.

LEG AND FOOT CRAMPS*

1. Relax twice a day in a tub of *warm* (not hot) water. Keep a spray running underwater, as you massage and manipulate feet and toes. Wash feet gently with a soft cloth and mild soap. After five minutes lift feet under warmer spray for a minute; then reimmerse in bath. Repeat six times.

2. Gently apply rubbing alcohol and dry thoroughly, but gently. Then gently massage with special ointment, diluted liniment, lanolin, cocoa butter, or oil. Dust on talcum powder.

3. Avoid extremes of temperature. Keep feet warm and dry. Change socks twice a day. At night wear loose-fitting bed socks.

4. Always wear properly fitted shoes with low heels and wide toes, of soft leather or lined with moleskin. (Do not wear rubber shoes or bedroom slippers or walk with bare feet.)

5. Once a week examine your feet and trim your toenails after washing. Cut straight across. For brittle nails apply lanolin and bandage loosely.

6. Do not cut corns, calluses, or ingrown nails. Have this done by your podiatrist.

7. Adhere to prescribed diet—high in protein, moderately low in fat, low in carbohydrate.

8. Do not use tobacco in any form.

9. If the skin is broken or inflamed, do not put weight on your leg; wash carefully and apply sterile, dry gauze. Never use antiseptics, iodine, Lysol, creosol, formaldehyde, or phenol preparations. If in doubt, consult your podiatrist. Cramps are an indication of vascular problems. When the blood supply is diminished to the lower extremities, the skin becomes thinner and more susceptible to abrasions, ulcers, and infections.

10. With foot swelling or previous phlebitis, elevate the foot of the bed 4 inches. When sitting, elevate legs on a stool.

11. Do not wear constricting garters or bandages. Do not cross your legs when sitting or standing for long periods. Keep off your feet for five minutes every hour; remove your shoes and massage and exercise your toes.

*Courtesy of Riker Laboratories, Inc., Northridge, California 91324.

Chapter 24
Lower Back Pain

Before you ask why I've included a small section on *backs* in a book about *feet,* you should know that even well-known runners like cardiologist/writer George Sheehan agree with me: 80 percent of lower back pain can be cured when you start from the ground up, at your feet.

Why Is Your Back So Directly Connected to Your Foot Pain?

Even though lower back pain can arise from disorders too numerous to list completely here—vascular disorders, neurological problems, tumors, cancer, kidney ailments—most of the time, something is wrong with the way you are standing, walking, and otherwise using your feet.

Your back is a very complex structure. Bones, joints, ligaments, and nerves all converging back there are incredibly sensitive to the shocks and bumps of simple movement. The disks which make up your backbone bear the brunt. If your spine is continually out of alignment, its muscular support has probably been compromised. Poor posture can change the length of your muscles, and when they're overstretched, they can't support you. You get dull muscle backaches.

How Do High Arches Cause an Aching Back?

If your arch is too high, it will send painful signals up to your lower back. This is because people with high arches have very heavy heel strikes. The ability to absorb shock in such a foot is limited, and so all the force each step carries is sent straight up your leg to your spine. What adds to the high-arch problem is the lack of extra padding or soft tissue on the heel. Obviously such a heel hasn't had much time to build support with all the shock it absorbs on a regular basis. The name for a foot with an extremely high arch is a *cavus foot*. If you look at the word *cavus*, you can clearly see the word *cave*. If you've got a cavus foot, your instep resembles a small cave. I've known patients who believed that their high-arched foot meant a good foot, but that isn't quite true, as I've already explained. The shock of your step is being unnaturally distributed to your heel and the ball of your foot and both these areas can end up sore. The pain can go all the way up to your lower back.

How Do You Treat This Problem?

If your high-arched foot puts you in pain, what a podiatrist does is treat the symptoms as they arise. Sometimes an orthotic placed under your arch works very well. And sometimes heel cups or padding across the metatarsal area of your foot redistributes the shock.

What About an Overly Pronated, or Uncomfortably Flat, Foot?

Excessive pronation of your feet can also cause lower back pain. A simple flat foot isn't the problem, as I've explained; it is the *pronation*, or the degree to which your arch sags each time you take a step, that causes the difficulties. When you have an overly pronated arch, your forefeet move too much when you walk. You are unbalanced, and this puts extra pressure on your muscles and joints and, of course, your lower back. High heels can be killers in this case. Your normal heel-to-toe movement is even more distorted, your pelvis will tilt forward, and if you wear heels constantly, the pelvic muscles will lose their tone.

What Happens If Your Legs Are
Slightly Different in Length?

If the difference is more than ¼ inch because of heredity or injury, your hips will tilt slightly and your spine may curve to one side or the other trying to correct the difference. Your center of gravity will be thrown off just below your navel and so will the muscles in your lower back. Since any imbalance in your body will be corrected at the bottom somewhere, you will end up with pain in your feet as well as your back.

Can a Bunion, a Painful Callus, or a Simple Ingrown Toenail
Give You Back Pain?

If you try to take the pressure off the painful area of your foot and throw your weight in the opposite direction, you can end up changing your gait. When you do this, you will be pushing muscles out of alignment. This will make them tire faster and hurt.

How Do You Treat Lower Back Pain When Your Feet Are
the Reason Your Back Hurts So Much?

Acute pain in the lower back can be alleviated with bed rest, analgesics, and physiotherapy. But to avoid a recurrence, feet should be examined for a biomechanical problem or abnormality that might be the cause. Many of my patients with lower back pain respond immediately to a combination of shoe orthotics and exercises to strengthen the back muscles. The orthotics help by absorbing some of the shock feet feel hitting the ground and by redistributing weight to correct the biomechanical imbalance. If the problem can be traced to a slight leg length difference, a small insert will be needed for the shoe of the shorter leg. Lower back pain almost always disappears immediately if this is the cause.

THE CASE OF THE HIGH-HEELED SLIPPER

When Gabrielle walked into my office that first time, I suspected the cause of her lower back pain. She obviously did too, or she would have been in the office of a back specialist and not a podiatrist.

Her occupation had created the crisis. She worked as a buyer in a very fashionable New York City department store. Days were spent on her feet, in high-heeled high-fashion footwear. The result: an aching back and severe pain in the balls or metatarsal arches of both feet. I suggested padding for her shoes in the metatarsal area. It didn't work. Her feet hurt even more. I prescribed flats. They only made matters worse. She had been wearing high heels so long that the cords of fiber at the back of her heel had become shortened and unable to stretch to accommodate flat shoes. The next thing I knew, the muscles in the backs of her legs were aching. And Gabrielle's abdominal muscles were also weak, so they weren't helping matters in the least.

Finally, Gabrielle agreed to wear shoes with a 1-inch heel to lengthen those heel and back-of-the-leg muscles, and she started on my prescribed exercise plan. We had found a plan to eliminate her pain at last.

What Kinds of Exercises Will Help Lower Back Pain?

The best exercise I know is the pelvic tilt. Lie on your back, with your knees slightly bent. Make sure you are on a fairly hard surface. A soft bed won't do. Now, press your lower back toward the floor. Flatten your back. Hold that position for ten seconds. Then relax. Repeat this for a few minutes each day.

It's a simple maneuver, but in the long run it will do worlds of good.

Riker Laboratories in Northridge, California, suggests nine other exercises in addition to the pelvic tilt. "Exercise for Better Back Care" is the same list I give to my patients.

Exercises for Better Back Care

General Instructions

Follow your doctor's instructions carefully. Start slowly and gradually increase speed and repetition. **Don't overdo it,** but exercise daily or not at all. The important thing is to relax. Exercise on a rug or mat. Put a pillow under your neck. Dress comfortably; no shoes or socks. Stop doing any exercise that causes pain until you have checked with your doctor.

1 Lie on your back with knees bent. Feet flat on the floor. Take a deep breath and relax. Press the small of your back against the floor and tighten your stomach and seat muscles. This should cause the lower end of the pelvis to rotate forward. Hold for five seconds. Relax. Repeat ten times.

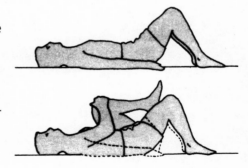

2 Lie on your back with knees bent. Feet flat on the floor. Take a deep breath and relax. Grasp **one** knee with both hands and pull it as close to your chest as possible. Return to starting position. Straighten leg. Return to starting position. Repeat ten times for each leg, alternating legs.

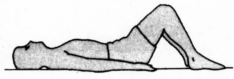

3 Lie on your back with knees bent. Feet on the floor. Take a deep breath and relax. Grasp **both** knees and pull them as close to your chest as possible. Return to starting position. Straighten legs. Return to starting position. Relax. Repeat ten times.

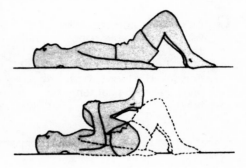

4 Lie on your back with knees bent. Feet flat on the floor. Take a deep breath and relax. Draw one knee to chest. Then point leg upward as far as possible. Return to starting position. Relax. Repeat ten times, alternating legs. *NOTE:* This exercise is not recommended for patients with sciatic pain.

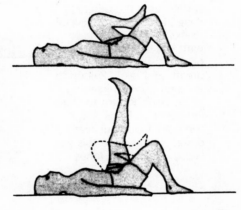

5 Lie on side with knees bent. Take a deep breath and relax. Slide upper knee toward chest as far as possible. Return to starting position. Relax. Repeat ten times on each side.

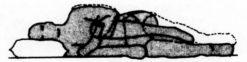

6 Lie on your stomach with your head on your hands. Take a deep breath and relax. Tighten your seat muscles. Hold for two seconds. Relax. Repeat ten times.

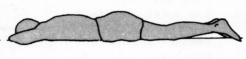

7 This exercise should not be started until the others have been done for several weeks. Lie on your back with knees bent. Feet flat on floor. Take a deep breath and relax. Pull up to a sitting position keeping knees bent. Return to starting position. Relax. Having someone hold your feet down can facilitate this exercise. Repeat ten times.

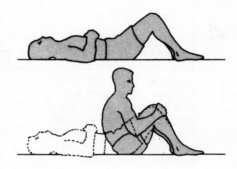

8 Lie on your back with your legs straight out, knees unbent and arms at your sides. Take a deep breath and relax. Raise legs one at a time as high as is comfortable and lower to floor as slowly as possible. Repeat five times for each leg.

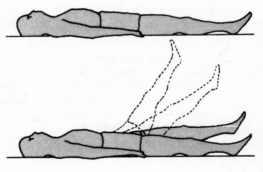

9 Get down on your hands and knees. Take a deep breath and relax. Pull stomach in and curve back upward. Let head hang down. Now arch back and look up. Relax. Repeat ten times.

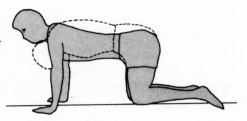

10 Stand with your back against doorway. Place heels 4 inches away from frame. Take a deep breath and relax. Press the small of your back against doorway. Tighten your stomach and seat muscles, allowing your knees to bend slightly. This should cause the lower end of the pelvis to rotate forward (as in exercise 1). Press your neck up against doorway. Press both hands against opposite side of doorway and straighten both knees. Hold for two seconds. Relax. Repeat ten times.

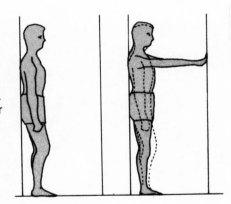

Helpful Hints for a Healthy Back

Always sit all the way back in a chair with your back erect. When you lift any object from the floor, bend your legs and keep your back straight; make your leg muscles do the work.

Sleep on a firm mattress or put a ¾-inch plywood board under a soft one. If you sleep on your back, put a pillow under your knees, not under your head. Keep your knees bent when sleeping on your side. Don't sleep on your stomach. When driving a car, keep the seat forward so your body is erect. On long trips, stop every hour or so and walk around to relieve tension and relax muscles.

When doing any work that requires standing, place one foot on a stool or bench. Be conscious of your posture, and avoid "sway" back. Tuck the pelvis forward to straighten the back. Walk whenever you get the chance. Once your backache is gone, get regular exercise and make a conscious effort to relax several times a day. If your back acts up, see your doctor immediately. Don't wait until it gets worse.

PART THREE
Love-Your-Feet Lessons

This last section is designed to take you past any immediate ache or pain into a lifelong program for understanding the signals feet send, and taking proper care of these two overworked parts of your body.

Chapter 25
Observe Your Lifestyle

Walk into any office and more likely than not, you'll see women's feet unobtrusively slipped out of their shoes. Glance down any city street and you'll see men making their way block after block wearing heavy, closed shoes in the middle of the summer. While there may be few people currently combining furs, silks, business suits, and sports sneakers, there aren't enough to suit the number of poor, neglected, underappreciated feet I see.

Patients come into my office all the time complaining and describing symptoms that come from the way they live. It doesn't seem to matter whether they are movers and shakers, semiactive exercisers, or sedentary slowpokes, their feet send them to see me. Their feet feel the pressures of their lifestyles. I've come up with three foot personalities along with the exercises and advice helpful for each. Whether you are the busy mother of a toddler or a runner on the New York Stock Exchange, the good news is that you can protect your feet and head off unpleasant problems before they plague you enough to go to a podiatrist.

The exercises and routines are not difficult, time-consuming, expensive, or equipment-oriented. In fact, you can do most of these anytime or anywhere without changing into leotards or special clothes. But just because they appear simple doesn't mean the rewards aren't plentiful.

Here are my three basic foot groups with the tips to keep your feet in tip-top shape.

The Sedentary Slowpoke

You prefer to sit and read the newspaper on Sunday morning. You've never considered jogging because your neighbors might notice you weren't in good shape when you set your two feet out the door. You do several sit-ups each morning and feel comfortable thinking that it's the closest you want to get to those total "workouts" described in the media. You want to lose a little weight, but food is too important. After all, you only live once, so why torture yourself? Who or what are you hurting anyway?

Your feet, that's what you are hurting! There's no need to feel guilty about your lifestyle, and I'm not suggesting you start running marathons. But even you would be surprised by how easy it is to incorporate a small dose of exercise into your routine. And how good you would feel all over.

Why Exercise?

The purpose of any exercise program is to maintain your body's flexibility and to keep your muscles stretched and working. When muscles and ligaments are being used daily, your joints will work properly. In a sense, if you neglect to "oil" your joints, they will "rust up" on you. Start by setting aside twenty minutes each day, or even less. But do start.

Start slowly. I am living proof of the value of this advice, for I was careless last winter when I went skiing for the first time in twelve years. I believed my body would be able to pick up where I left off more than a decade before. And though my nerve didn't fail me, my lack of conditioning did. Three weeks after my skiing adventure, I still had a swollen left ankle from a sprain that could easily have been avoided.

Where to Begin to Put Your Feet and Ankles in Order First?

The Foot Press

This exercise is essential for strengthening the muscles in your feet that have become slack from sitting so much. It's also marvelous for your arches and ankles, and your thighs may tighten too.

First take your shoes off. Cross your legs at the ankles and keep one foot on top of the other. Now try pulling them away from each other and really put the pressure on. Next, sit down on the floor and bend your legs at the knees, putting the soles of your feet together. Press them against one another and hold the pose for at least two minutes.

Five Desk Dares

Place a phone book on the floor, slip off your shoes, and curl your toes over the edges of the pages. As your flexibility increases, you'll gradually be able to ripple the pages. This is a great exercise for fighting foot fatigue and for strengthening the muscles of your feet.

Start with an empty bottle, or a handful of pencils, or some marbles under your desk. Roll your shoeless feet over them. This will stimulate the blood flow in sedentary feet. The back-and-forth motion acts like a massage.

Play pick-up-sticks with your toes and don't cheat. Grasp a stick or a marble or a pencil with your toes to stretch ligaments and loosen tight toes.

If your office is semiprivate, place your feet on a pedestal or on top of your desk. Elevating them several times a day—even for a moment or two—will stimulate circulation. You can actually feel the blood rush from your feet, and for me, it's an instant relief.

Take off your shoes and write the letters of the alphabet using your toes. Seriously, it's a great trick. If you are at home, have the kids try it too. Do A to Z with one foot, and then start with the other.

More Suggestions for Sedentaries

- If you are in the habit of sitting at a desk during your lunch break, break it. Bring or wear that pair of sneakers to work and start putting them on at lunchtime. Twenty city blocks are approximately equal to 1 mile so even ten blocks will start you off in the right direction. And because walking may stimulate the production of endorphins, chemicals in your body which may make you feel less hungry, you could end up eating less at lunch and losing weight.

* Having two pairs of shoes on hand during your daily routine is a good idea for more reasons than exercise. Women suffer four times more foot problems than men because they wear shoes with pointy toes and high heels. Simply by varying the styles during the course of a single day, you offer your imprisoned foot more breathing room. You guard against inflaming a bunion and protect yourself from pump bumps on your heel. Changing shoe heights will also stretch your heel cords so you'll be exercising your feet without effort. Width changes make a difference too. Slipping into the narrow toe box of dressy shoes after having your toes spread wide in sneakers may change the way your foot receives the pressure of walking.

The Semiactive Exerciser

You spend a lot of your life on your feet or if not actually up and about, you certainly move around a lot. You exercise fairly regularly. You are energetic and think you should be doing more. But you probably can't find the time because of children, work, friends, and lovers or other strangers. Nevertheless, whether you are the mother of a busy toddler, a salesperson, or a cop on a walking beat, your feet are going to feel the stress of your physical life. You need to listen to the signals they send you even more than the sedentary slowpoke. It has been calculated that you are putting about 700 tons of weight on your feet in the course of a day. If you are a salesperson or a stewardess, the weight is even worse. If this is the case, I often recommend that individuals try to change the position in which they stand or the way they walk, as well as the shoes they wear.

Why Do You Feel Like Shifting Your Weight When You Stand Still Too Long?

When all your body's weight is being transmitted to your feet standing in a single position, your bones are actually more susceptible to injury. Why? Because the soft tissue on the soles of your feet is receiving constant pressure. Can you remember the last time you stood in line for a movie and had to keep shifting your weight from one foot to the other? It's not an accident that you were compelled to do so. Your feet were crying out to be relieved of some of this pressure. They weren't designed to hold up a statue.

If you live a life that demands that you stay on your feet all day, try crepe-soled shoes and do stay away from high heels. Try putting a piece of soft carpeting under your feet. The bare floor under your feet may be too much for your feet to bear. Even the healthy, active person can't stand in one position endlessly without agony.

Inside Insight for the Semiactives

- The next time you are standing or waiting, come up on your toes and then slip back down to your heels. This rocking motion redistributes the pressure you are inflicting on your feet.
- Walk on the outside of your feet. Alternately, rest your weight on that outside edge, one at a time to avoid twisting your ankles.
- Climb the walls! Lie on your back, and let your feet walk up the sides of the nearest wall. It builds strength and is great for your circulation.
- I call this one the *toe-heel*. Take off your shoes and stretch your feet for a minute wiggling all your toes at the same time. Now, walk across the room on your toes. (Don't try to be a ballet star. En pointe is not necessary for a full stretch.) Coming back, lean back and walk on your heels.
- If you are the mother of children, you'll love the *stretch*. Have one of your children lie down beside you. Sesame Street or Romper Room is a fine accompaniment. Find a comfortable spot on the floor, shoes off, lie flat on your back. Now, lift your legs up until they are at right angles to your body. Point your toes to the ceiling. Feel that stretch from the front of your ankle to the tip of your toes. Reverse and push your heel up now. Hold each pose for at least sixty seconds.
- The *swollen ankle cure* is great for anyone who has put too much pressure on his or her feet and ended up with a stiffened, swollen extremity as a result. Find a comfortable spot on the floor, take off your shoes and choose between sitting or lying down. It doesn't matter much. Now, flex both feet so they are flat on the floor. Make the stretch travel up to your knees. These ligaments and muscles are

rarely given this kind of opportunity. To stretch the ligaments and muscles up the back of your leg, press you knees into the floor flat. Now, ease up on your flexing, lean over, and pull your feet toward you slightly, pulling on the balls. Keep your legs straight for the full effect and try to keep your back flat too.

• The *ankle extra* may work wonders at times. Lying on the floor on your back, lift one leg at a time into the air. Circle the raised foot in one direction and then the other. Try to keep each leg up for at least sixty seconds per leg. Make your leg stay at least 2 inches off the floor, if not higher. The idea is to keep the leg above the level of your heart so your blood will flow faster back to the heart as opposed to away from it. This is a good exercise for the thighs, too.

Word of Warning for Weekend Athletes: You are the most frequent victims of overexertion due to underconditioning. Muscles, tendons, ligaments, bones, and joints can all become injured or inflamed from sudden abuse.

The Mover and Shaker

You have run marathons and intend to do so again. You bicycle up to 30 miles at a time. You swim. You belong to a health club and go at least once a day. You are certainly physically fit. But every once in a while, and sometimes more than you care to admit, your feet pay the price for your high-powered schedule.

Though disciplined exercisers are obviously in shape and can often take more foot abuse than anyone else, they run the risk of more acute foot injury. Consider this: the feet of a 6-foot-tall, 200-pound marathon runner who moves in 1-yard strides will absorb a total of 352,000 pounds of stress for each mile run. Type-three people rarely run only one mile, so, they put a lot of pressure on their feet.

Of late, ailments have been named for athletic pursuits which have made them increasingly common: "tennis toe" and "jogger's knee," for example. Other common and acute problems are blisters, arch troubles, shin splints, and disappearing toe nails.

Tips for Movers and Shakers

- Slip off your shoes to *pump the gas pedal,* or make sure your shoes are fairly flat. Sitting down, simply pretend that you are pumping the gas pedal with your right foot and then the left. This will exercise your ankle as well as the muscles in your feet.
- An uncomplicated calisthenic for especially limber individuals is the *balancing act.* Hang your briefcase or pocketbook or some other weight over the top of your foot. Be sure you can hold onto the weight for several minutes. Now, in a sitting position, raise your foot, bend your leg at the knee, and bring the weight toward you.
- Never dismiss the value of stretching. Your legs are controlled by muscles that work in opposition to each other. The stronger muscle may cause the weaker one to tear or strain. In order to figure out which muscles need more stretching, picture them in a split body. The muscles in the front of your body are called the antigravity muscles and are often weaker than the ones in the back of your body. These two groups are constantly interacting with each other, contracting and lengthening each other.
- Do the stretching exercises described in the next section.

EXERCISE #1

Front Thigh Stretch (Standing)

(Quadriceps Femoris and Hip Flexor Group)

Starting Position: Stand on a firm surface with one arm holding onto a chair or a wall for support and stability (Exercise #1A).

Action: With the free hand grasp the instep of the foot and bring the heel of the foot inward toward your buttocks. When you experience a stretching sensation in the front portion of the thigh, hold the leg at that position (Exercise #1B) for thirty seconds, relax for fifteen seconds, and repeat the stretch for thirty seconds. NOTE: You should be standing straight up throughout the entire exercise.

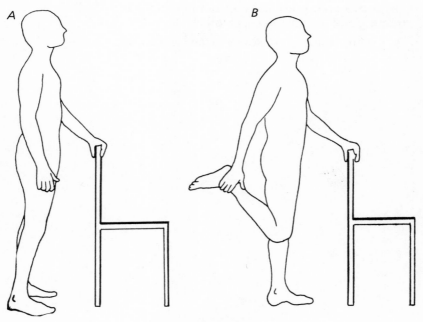

Exercise #1

EXERCISE #2

Front Thigh Stretch On a Table

(Quadriceps Femoris and Hip Flexor Group)

Starting Position: Lie down on your back on a table with the leg that has to be exercised hanging over the side of the table (Exercise #2A).

Action: Grasp the instep of the foot and bring the heel of the foot in the direction of the buttocks. When you experience a stretching sensation in the front portion of the thigh, hold the leg at that position (Exercise #2B).

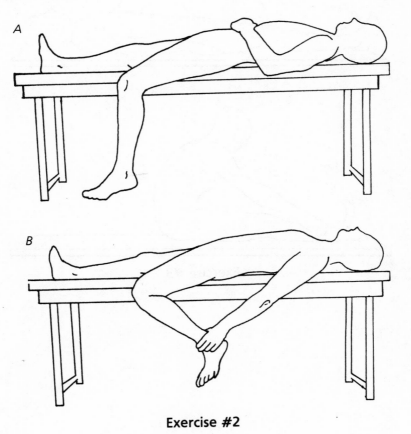

Exercise #2

EXERCISE #3

Posterior Thigh Stretching—Supine Position

**(Sacrospinalis, Gluteus Maximus, Hamstrings,
and Triceps Surae Group)**

Starting Position and Action: Lie down on your back on the floor
(Exercise #3A). Bring the front portion of your body up over the legs
until you experience a stretching sensation in the posterior portion of
your legs. Hold that position by grasping the legs (Exercise #3B). NOTE:
Make sure both legs remain straight throughout the exercise.

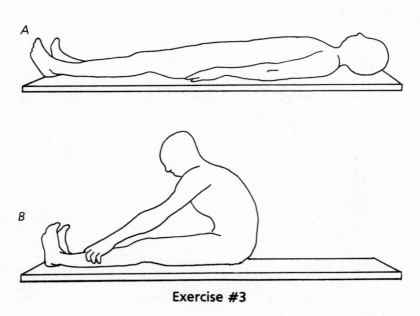

Exercise #3

EXERCISE #4

Posterior Thigh Stretching Seated On a Table

(Sacrospinalis, Gluteus Maximus, Hamstrings, and Triceps Surae Group)

Starting Position: Stand alongside a table; place the leg that has to be exercised on the long axis of the table (Exercise #4A).

Action: Bend the "standing leg" at the knee until you experience a slight stretching sensation in the posterior portion of the thigh that is on the table. Hold that position. Bring the front portion of the body over the legs again, until you experience the stretching sensation in the posterior portion of the legs. Hold that position by grasping the legs (Exercise #4B). NOTE: To stretch the calf muscles, point the toes upward and toward your chest.

A   B

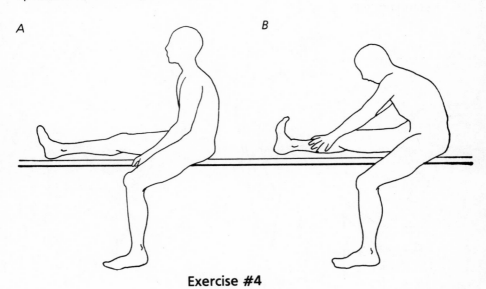

Exercise #4

EXERCISE #5

Posterior Thigh Stretching—Standing Position

(Sacrospinalis, Gluteus Maximus, Hamstrings, and Triceps Surae Group)

Starting Position: Stand in front of a table. Place the leg that has to be exercised on the table (Exercise #5A).

Action: Bend the standing leg at the knee until you experience a slight stretching sensation in the posterior portion of the thigh that is on the table. Holding that position, *bring the front portion* of the body over the legs until you experience the stretching sensation in the posterior portion of the legs. Hold that position by grasping the leg (Exercise #5B). To stretch the calf muscles, point the toes toward your chest. NOTE: If you have a disability in both legs, *do not* bend the standing leg.

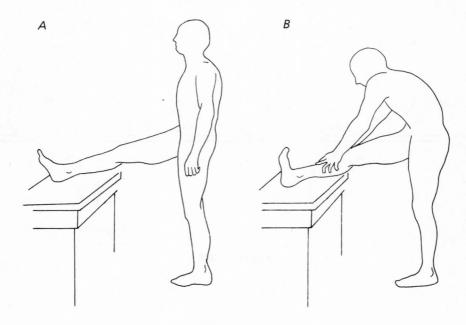

A   B

Exercise #5

EXERCISE #6

Posterior Thigh Stretching—Standing Position

(Sacrospinalis, Gluteus Maximus, Hamstrings, and Triceps Surae Group)

Starting Position: Stand to the side of a table; place the leg that has to be exercised on the table (Exercise #6A). Turn the entire leg inward such that the inside portion of your foot is facing the table.

Action: Bend the standing leg at the knee until you experience a slight stretching sensation in the posterior portion of the thigh on the table. Holding that position, *bring the side of your body* over the legs until you experience the stretching sensation in the posterior portion of the legs. Hold that position by grasping the leg (Exercise #6B). To stretch the calf muscles, point the toes toward your chest. Repeat the exercise with your feet turned outward one at a time. NOTE: If you have a disability in both legs *do not* bend the standing leg.

A   B

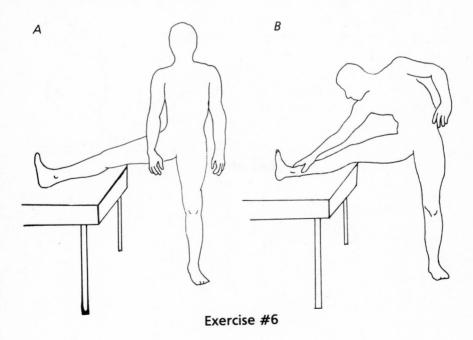

Exercise #6

EXERCISE #7

Inner Thigh Stretch—Sitting Position

Starting Position: Sitting on a floor, place the soles of your feet together and bring them in toward the buttocks (Exercise #7A).
Action: From the starting position, place the hands on the knees and push the knees down toward the floor (Exercise #7B).

A

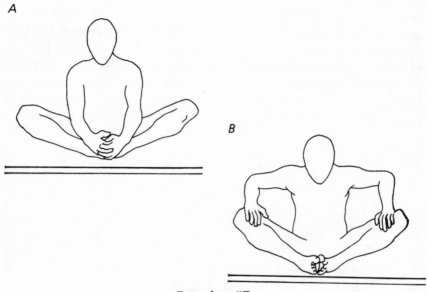

B

Exercise #7

EXERCISE #8

Calf Stretch

(Triceps Surae Group)

Starting Position: Stand two feet away from a wall or as far away as you can before you begin to feel a pull in the muscle. Place the palms of your hands against the wall (Exercise #8A).

Action: From the starting position, lean your body in toward the wall (by bending the shoulders, elbows, and wrists) until you feel a stretching sensation in the back of the calf muscles (Exercise #8B). NOTE: Make sure the body is kept straight throughout the entire exercise, and that the heels remain on the ground.

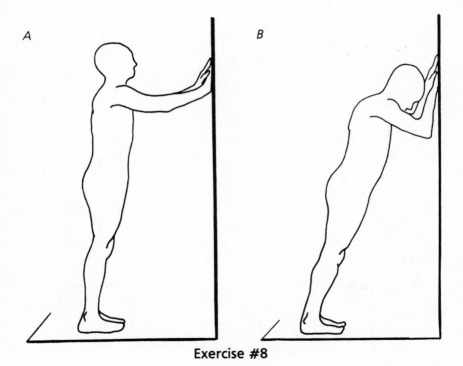

A   B

Exercise #8

EXERCISE #9

Calf Stretch

(Triceps Surae Group)

Starting Position: Standing with both feet on a step, footstool, or chair, place the ball of the foot that has to be exercised on the edge (Exercise #9A).

Action: From the starting position push the heel that has to be stretched below the level of the footstool until you begin to feel a stretch in the calf muscles. To increase the stretch, bend the other leg at the knee (Exercise #9B).

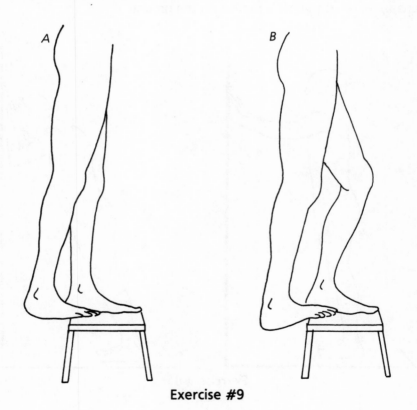

Exercise #9

EXERCISE #10

Calf Stretch

(Soleus Muscle)

Starting Position: In a standing position, place the foot that has to be exercised flat on a chair or footstool (Exercise #10A).
Action: Keeping the heel down, lean your body over the chair or footstool until you feel a stretching sensation in the back of the calf (Exercise #10B).

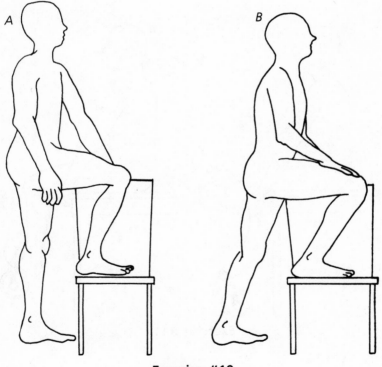

Exercise #10

EXERCISE #11

Ankle Dorsiflexion

(Tibialis Anterior Group)

Starting Position: Sit on the edge of a high desk or table with the knees bent and the weights above the level of the floor (Exercise #11A). Secure the weights around the instep of the foot.

Exercise: Bring the toes up toward the front of the leg by bending the ankle (Exercise #11B). Perform this exercise twenty-five times, relax for thirty seconds, then repeat twenty-five times for a total of fifty repetitions.

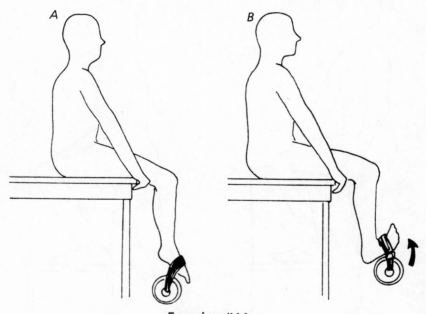

Exercise #11

EXERCISE #12

Ankle Inversion

(Tibialis Posterior Group)

Starting Position: Lie down on the side of your body with the foot to be exercised; the foot should be positioned off the edge of the table, below the ankle bone. Secure weights around the instep of the foot (Exercise #12A).

Exercise: Turn the ankle so that the toes face up toward the ceiling (Exercise #12B). Perform the exercise twenty-five times, relax for thirty seconds; then repeat twenty-five times for a total of fifty repetitions.

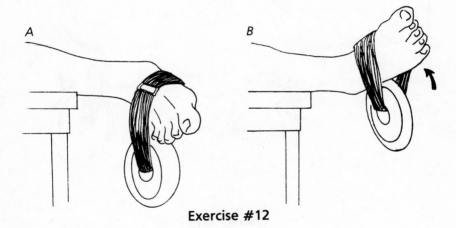

Exercise #12

EXERCISE #13

Ankle Eversion

(Peroneal Group)

Starting Position: Lie down with the side of your body with the foot to be exercised on top; the foot should be positioned off the edge of the table. Secure weights around the instep of the foot (Exercise #13A).

Exercise: Turn the ankle upward, raising the toes as high as possible (Exercise #13B). Perform the exercise twenty-five times; relax for thirty seconds; repeat twenty-five times for a total of fifty repetitions.

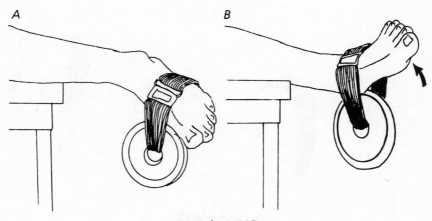

Exercise #13

EXERCISE #14

Ankle Plantar Flexion

(Triceps Surae Group)

Starting Position: Place a 1-inch book or a board of similar thickness under the front of the foot to be exercised. The other leg is bent at the knee so that its foot is off the ground. Hold onto a chair or wall for added support (Exercise #14A).

Exercise: Push off the ball of the foot you are exercising by lifting the heel off the ground (Exercise #14B). Perform this motion twenty-five times, relax thirty seconds, then repeat twenty-five times for a total of fifty repetitions. NOTE: As the leg strengthens, increase the height of the book or board from 1 to 2 inches.

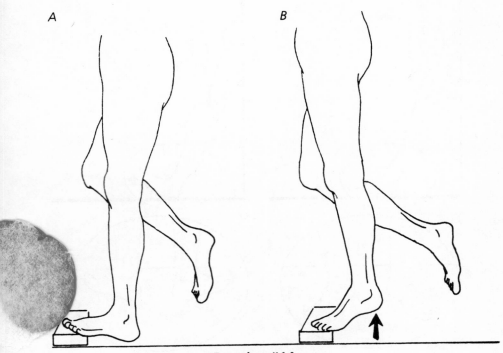

A   *B*

Exercise #14

EXERCISE #15

Ankle Eversion

(Peroneal Group)

Starting Position: Lean your back against a wall with both feet outwardly rotated and placed 12 inches in front of you (Exercise #15A).
Exercise: With the heels of your feet remaining on the ground, lift both feet up in the air (Exercise #15B).

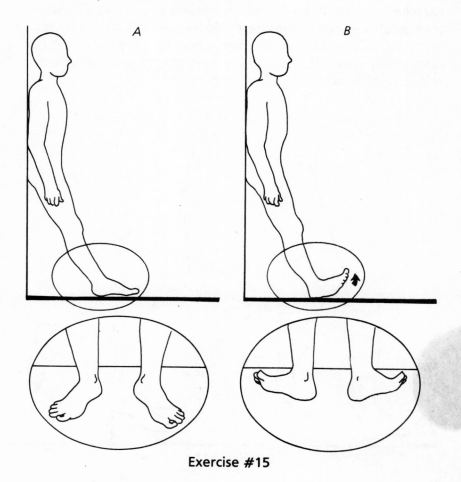

Exercise #15

A Word about Walking

Walking is one of the easiest, safest, and most natural ways to exercise. Henry David Thoreau thought walkers were a class apart. The poet Wadsworth walked 14 miles a day.

If you are beginning a walking program to get into better shape, keep in mind that a stroll will not give you the same results that a brisk pace will. As you walk to stay fit, all of the muscles in your body—in your feet, your buttocks, your thighs, abdomen, diaphragm, and upper torso—will be alternately contracting and relaxing. A vigorous walk will strengthen your heart and your circulation and tone your muscles.

Good News for Walkers

A recent study of 1200 joggers done by the United States Centers for Disease Control found that one out of four suffered some injury to their muscles and bones and one out of every seven had been to a doctor recently for injuries. But the center reported rare catastrophes to walkers.

Chapter 26
Children's Feet

Most people would agree that there is nothing more beautiful than the simple perfection of a baby's hands and feet. I often hear adults marveling that baby's feet are such perfect miniatures. But while babies' feet may look like replicas of our own, they are actually very different in structure.

When you compare x-rays of a baby and an adult foot, it looks as if the baby's foot has many more bones than the adult foot. That's because the foot bones are not completely formed until a person is about 20 years old! Until that time, gaps of cartilage remain between the bones.

In all the intricacies of bone and cartilage that make up a baby's foot is the potential for a host of problems to develop and become the plagues of adult feet. But if treated with care, children's feet can be trouble-free feet for the rest of their walking lives.

Baby Basics

As a school project, a college athlete once attempted for an entire day to mimic the movements and actions of a small child.

As he soon found out, it's not as easy as it sounds! In fact, some contortions that are perfectly natural—and comfortable—for toddlers are nearly impossible for our adult frames. So we podiatrists need a whole separate vocabulary to describe kids' walking problems. And before we can assess any abnormalities, we need to know what's normal for youngsters of different ages.

To give you an idea of the common stages that children go through, here are some general guidelines based on my own observations:

- Until they are about two years old, children are commonly bow-legged. (A note of caution, however: Don't overdo it with double-diapering. Too much bulkiness can force a child's legs into an even more extreme outward position.)
- When first starting to walk, most kids take a wide stance, holding their arms out for more stability.
- From ages two to four, many children become knock-kneed.
- Four- to six-year-olds are commonly bowlegged.
- In girls, bowleggedness may last until they are about eight years old.

Many parents have also consulted me because they were concerned that their babies had flat feet. Let me say that this is a perfectly normal condition. Babies' feet almost always look flat until they are two or three years old. The reason they look flat is not a deformity of the arch, as parents naturally worry, but a fat pad that spontaneously disappears once the child begins to walk. A visible arch usually develops with walking by about the age of four. If the feet *are* abnormally flat and if treatment by a podiatrist is necessary, it will still be very effective after the child turns four, so there's really no cause for alarm before that time.

Creative Correctives

Many of the differences that make your child's feet unique are no more dangerous than differences in hair color or facial shape. But there are some flaws that can become problems in later life if left untreated. I've compiled a list of the foot maladies I see most often in kids, along with my own recommended course of action in each case.

Overlapping Toes   About one out of every four babies has a toe that overlaps or underlaps its next-door neighbor. This occurs quite commonly when the fifth toe—the "baby" toe—overlaps the fourth, or when the second toe overlaps the third. Taping the toes into the correct position using adhesive tape can effectively eliminate the problem if it's done conscientiously when the child is between the ages of six months and one year. Taping can also help to rectify a toe that is not completely straight, but in both cases, the taping must be done *very* regularly for it to have the desired effect. If neglected, crooked or overlapping toes may have to be surgically corrected later in life.

Toeing In, Toeing Out   Most babies first learning to walk will turn their toes in or out a little bit. In those first awkward months, these toeing-in or toeing-out positions add some stability to a toddler's walk. Generally, kids will outgrow this by the time they are about seven or eight. If the problem persists, it's a good idea to have a doctor evaluate the child's walk.

If you're worried because your child's feet seem to point unusually inward or outward, I recommend that you trust your instincts as a parent and take your child to see a podiatrist. Even though most toeing-in or -out problems I've seen have been relatively harmless, there are occasional instances where a severely turned stance will cause damage to the foot or will cause the arch to collapse from constant pressure that the arch can't handle. In these cases, a podiatrist can examine the child to find out what is causing the toeing in or out. If it is being caused by too-tight muscular contraction in the legs, most doctors (myself included) will recommend a night splint—usually called a "bar"—for your child. (In kids whose outward or inward rotation is caused by a bone deformity, a bar probably won't help—and may even hurt. Only a doctor can evaluate the cause and prescribe the right corrective.) You'll find that most children get used to sleeping with a bar within a day or two, and in my experience the results have been very good.

There are other things you can do to help circumvent more serious rotation problems. As I'm sure you're aware, lots of children have a habit of sitting on their own feet while they're playing or watching television. Take a closer look next time you see your child doing this. Many times this activity forces a child's feet into even more extreme toeing in or out. It's best to discourage this kind of sitting as much as possible.

With babies, if a bar isn't prescribed, I suggest that you subtly supervise your child's sleeping position. First watch how your baby normally sleeps. Chances are, sleeping babies will exaggerate the toeing in or out that's natural for them when awake. The best way I've found to prevent this is to prop them up on their side with a pillow to keep them from sleeping on their stomach. Most parents I've given this suggestion to have found that it works—and with very few complaints from the little one.

A note of caution: Toeing out is sometimes a symptom of another problem—weak arches. This is actually the most common foot problem in young children, but if left untreated, it can cause a wide range of side effects later in life. It's sad for me to see adults with poor posture, awkward gaits, lower back pain, or leg cramping that could have been avoided if they had been treated for a relatively minor arch problem at a young-enough age. In cases in which children have extreme inward or outward leg roatation, I'd say it's best to let a podiatrist decide whether or not treatment is needed.

Knock-Knees or Bowlegs　　One of my favorite stories is about two little girls who were waiting in my office one day. One of the girls was bowlegged and the other was slightly knock-kneed. When I came in, they were standing side by side giggling, because they had just discovered that by standing next to each other, they could spell out the word *ox.*

Many years ago, knock-knees or bowlegs were usually symptoms of a nutritional problem, e.g., rickets. But these days such problems are increasingly rare, and most cases of knee deviation in either direction will correct themselves as the child reaches the age of eight.

Other Problems

Below, I've listed some other foot ailments that are common to children and what they generally signify:

Tiptoeing Around   Children just learning to walk who step mainly on their tiptoes may have shortened muscles in the backs of their legs. This problem is correctible but requires a visit to the doctor.

Sole problems   Mild clubfoot is an inherited condition that causes a baby's feet to look flat. You can distinguish between this and the "fat pads" I describe earlier in this chapter because with clubfoot there are noticeable wrinkles underneath the ankle-bone at the outside of the foot—even when the foot isn't bearing any weight. If untreated, these feet will become permanently flat and will probably cause problems later on.

Limping   There are four underlying causes I've discovered for children's limps, and in most cases a podiatrist is needed to determine the true problem in each case. First, a limp can be the result of an injury, ranging in severity from a blister to a cut or fracture. Second, heel problems or problems with the Achilles tendon may require a professional eye. Third, a wart, corn, or callus can be causing the child to limp. Fourth, and least common, are neurological diseases and legs of different lengths.

Warts, Corns, and Calluses   All of these appear in children with some frequency. The most important thing to remember about treating corns and calluses is that they are growths that signify another underlying problem. Usually by examining your child and asking a few key questions, a podiatrist can determine what is causing the problem. Warts are quite common in children and teenagers, as well, and need to be treated *before* they multiply or spread to the hands. In the meantime, I recommend that your youngster refrain from sharing socks, towels, or slippers with other children to avoid spreading the warts.

Leg Cramps   Kids between the ages of two and five often experience severe leg cramps at night. For years, doctors called them "growing pains" and considered them a normal occurrence. Now we realize that there are many potential reasons for this cramping and that cramps *can* be avoided. Fatigue, foot or leg strain, lowering the temperature of the house during the night, loss of adequate blood circulation (which can be as simple as sleeping with one leg crossed over the other), and a faulty gait may all be contributing factors. To relieve the pain momentarily, try massaging the cramped area. To prevent cramping, try to maintain an even temperature in the bedroom during the night. See a podiatrist if the problem persists.

Examining Your Baby at Home

After asking whether her baby is a girl or boy, one of the first questions a mother usually asks is, "Does she have all her fingers and toes?" While having all ten toes is certainly an important concern, I'd have to say that lack of them is the least common foot ailment afflicting young children.

After your baby has been home from the hospital long enough to adjust to the new surroundings, but while he or she is still an infant, try spotting any potential foot and leg problems by using the two methods I describe below.

- Lay the baby face up with knees together and hips and knees bent. In this position, the feet should point straight ahead and the legs should form parallel lines. Many common tendencies, such as toeing in, toeing out, bowleggedness, or knock-knees will be readily apparent in this position.
- The other good test is to lay your baby face down and look for any noticeable differences between the right and left buttocks. Are the

creases underneath the buttocks even? Is there a discrepancy between the two creases, along with one buttock being flatter and wider
than the other? If so, describe the differences to your pediatrician
to see if a doctor's examination is needed.

Walking Tall

It's common among parents to want their baby to reach every
milestone—smiling, cooing, walking, and talking—before the
official charts say she or he should. While this is perfectly natural, I will reassure you that there's *no* reason to worry if your
child is slightly behind the timetables. What *is* important is not
to force your child to walk before she or he is ready. Dangling
a baby by the armpits to try and get him or her to take the first
steps may strain muscles—and probably won't have him or her
walking any sooner.

I've included a timetable with the *approximate* ages and the
stages that your baby will go through on the road to walking.
It's meant to be a guideline, not a set of hard-and-fast rules, so
unless your child is more than three to six months behind this
schedule, don't let it worry you.

First Steps:

6 months	Crawling attempts
8 months	Tries to stand
12 months	Stands alone
14 months	Tries to walk
18 months	Walks alone comfortably
24 months	Runs
36 months	Runs, jumps, rarely stumbles

When your child first attempts to stand, if you have a playpen,
renovate it by covering the mattress with a soft blanket, tucked
in around all sides. I've found that this makes an ideal surface
for a child's tender feet to grasp, while also providing ample
warmth.

First Shoes

I understand the temptation to dress your baby in all the adorable little shoes and booties you've inevitably received as presents. However, it's essential that your baby's feet have room to move, and any foot covering provides unnecessary restrictions.

The only reason to cover your baby's feet is for warmth. Whether you dress your child in an all-in-one outfit or in separate socks, they should be made of cotton and should be woven so that there is enough width across the toes. Still, you must watch because the garment might shrink . . . and your baby might grow!

It's equally important to give your baby plenty of footroom when asleep. Try to avoid tucking in blankets too tightly. If tucking in is necessary for warmth, it will help to place a thick roll of diapers or extra blankets underneath the cover at the foot of the crib. This will keep the blanket loose over your baby's feet.

Only If the Shoe Fits

Many parents think it's necessary to put high-top shoes on their children at a very young age. My belief is that until babies are ready to stand, they are better off barefoot. And while high-tops are fine, they are *not* necessary for ankle support. Children need to develop strength in their ankles without any additional support. The benefits of high-tops are that they do not slip off as easily as low-cut shoes and that they help keep the ankles warm. And since leather high-tops cost much more than sneakers, they may not be the best investment for shoes that need to be replaced so frequently.

Sizing Them Up

Since no two feet are exactly the same size, I recommend having both of your child's feet measured when buying shoes and then fitting the larger foot. The Footwear Council recommends buying shoes that leave ¼ to ½ inch of space between the largest toe and the end of the shoe. Check to make sure that the shoes are deep enough at the toes not to press down on your child's feet and that the widest part of the shoe coincides with the ball of the foot.

Don't buy your child new shoes on a *regular* basis because the simple fact is, children's feet don't grow with any regularity. Often, there's a spurt of growth followed by a period where they grow very little. The best way to tell when your child needs new shoes is to check them for fit every few weeks.

Take a look at the chart I've included, provided by the Footwear Council. While it won't help—and may even hurt—to follow it exactly, it should give you an idea of the frequency with which you'll need to replace your child's shoes.

Age in Years	Size-Change Intervals
2 to 6	1 to 2 months
6 to 10	2 to 3 months
10 to 12	3 to 4 months
12 to 15	4 to 5 months
15 to 20	6 months

If the Shoe Doesn't Fit!

Here are some other signs which might be helpful in detecting an improper fit:

- Frequent pulling off of shoes. Many times I've found that children who take off their shoes at every opportunity are wearing shoes that don't fit correctly. Examine the shoes when your child is standing in them to make sure there's enough room, and check feet for blisters or other irritations.

- Red marks on the feet. These are created by pressure or friction and should be investigated.

- Sweating. Feet that sweat excessively may be strained. Check your child's socks at the end of the day to see if they are damp; it may mean that the muscles are working too hard to compensate for a misaligned foot.

- Heel pain. Active children between the ages of seven and twelve, particularly kids who are overweight, may experience soreness at the base of the Achilles tendon. This could signal bursitis or tendinitis. Temporarily refraining from exercise—particularly bicycling, which pulls on the heel—may help. Soaking the foot in hot water usually helps to ease the pain.

• Unevenly worn soles. Soles that are excessively worn on the outside heel are probably no cause for alarm. Figure 26-1 indicates the normal direction of weight-bearing forces. On the other hand, soles that are heavily worn on the instep may indicate foot or ankle problems that need to be examined.

A final word of advice: please don't pass on used shoes from one child to another. It may be tempting because kids rarely wear out their shoes by the time they outgrow them. But children's feet are so malleable that it's just not worth the potential harm.

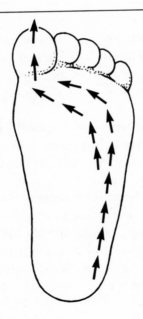

Figure 26-1
Normal direction of the weight-bearing forces through the foot.

Chapter 27
Aging Feet

"Grow old along with me, the best is yet to be," may be true for romance, but decidedly not for feet.

As a podiatrist, I may be prejudiced, but in no other part of your anatomy is your age more dramatically reflected than in your feet.

I remember the seventy-four-year-old golfer who played at least three times a week. She came to see me because of pain that suddenly made it impossible for her to walk as well as she had before. She was bright, alert, and wholly active—except for one painful foot. She also believed that once you were past fifty years of age, no corrective procedure should be done.

When I examined her, I found the big toe joint was stiff, barely moveable, and made a loud crackling noise when pushed. A painful bunion made the toe look even more twisted. Our treatment plan included surgical revision of the foot, with excision of the bunion. All surgery was done under a local anesthetic. Immediately after surgery, she was able to walk, and was quickly back in her normal shoes and on the golf course once more.

Aging feet, like this golfer's, present special problems. Changes in your feet are a result of the normal aging process, but they also may be the first signs of a more serious problem, such as diabetes, vascular disease, arthritis, or a degenerative joint disease. So it's important to keep on top of any discomfort. In a sense, as you grow older, you'll want to stay "on your toes."

The damage from years of wearing ill-fitting shoes, skin problems, corns, calluses, and brittle, bruised nails are seen more often in senior citizens. If you are over fifty, and your feet are killing you, it is well worth the time and money to have a careful foot examination, since you are more susceptible to infections, fractures, toenail changes, and biomechanical deformities like bunions and hammertoes. It might even be a musculoskeletal problem that began as a weak muscle somewhere else, or a limb length discrepancy.

The most common problems I see in older patients are ones I've already talked about, but it might be helpful to list them again: calluses, dry skin, and toenail troubles stand out.

What Are the Most Common Nail Problems in Older Feet?

Thickened toenails and ingrown toenails. If you have a thickened nail, you may think there is a corn under the nail that needs "cleaning out." This isn't true. Gradual thickening of the nail (onychauxis) is caused by repeated trauma, poor nutrition, and a change in circulation. Sometimes, after a long period of small but repeated injuries, as from poorly fitting shoes, your nail becomes thickened and discolored. Fungal infections can turn nails brown or yellowish. I've seen nails so brittle and cracked that they could even be peeled off.

How Can Ingrown Toenails Cause Problems?

When the nail grows down into the flesh, the flesh becomes irritated and an infection can begin (paronychia). Sometimes an abscess occurs. Incision, drainage, and removal of a piece of the nail, along with soaking and sometimes the use of antibiotics, are the best treatments for a neglected abscess. Sometimes so-called proud flesh, or red, sore tissue, accompanies repeated paronychia.

The most common causes of ingrown toenails are improper cutting of the nails and shoes that are too narrow. Some people are so eager to remove the grooves filled with "callus" that they end up cutting the sides of the nail, removing the part of the nail that meets the flesh. If your shoes are too narrow, they may squeeze the toes, causing the nail to grow into the flesh over time, particularly if you wear narrow shoes.

What Can You Do to Avoid Nail Problems?

First, avoid trauma to your toenails by refusing to wear shoes that don't fit. Next, cut your nails straight across and keep them short (Figure 27-1). It is also helpful to keep the nails clean by using a nail brush daily. Warm, soapy water can do wonders for dirt under the nails. If your feet perspire heavily, change your shoes often, and use a dusting of cornstarch to eliminate excess perspiration, which can provide the perfect breeding ground for fungal infections.

If you can't cut your own toenails easily or correctly, go to a physician. Don't allow a nail to separate from its bed, because this forms a perfect setting for a bacterial or fungal infection, and it could be more dangerous than you think.

If these steps don't work, a troublesome nail can be removed by your physician, using a local anesthetic injected into the

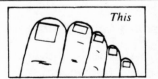 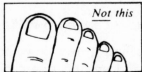

Figure 27-1
How to cut a toenail. Cut your nails straight across. Do not cut into the corners and do not cut close to the flesh.

base of your toe. If you don't have circulation problems, the base of the nail can be surgically removed or chemically cauterized so a deformed nail won't grow back again.

How Can Sudden Trauma Cause Nail Problems?

Tripping and striking the toe, injuring the nail plate, happens all the time, and is a direct result of an unsteady gait that aging and some systemic problems can bring.

If this happens to you, and you are concerned about the pain, you should have your toe x-rayed to see if it has been fractured. If not, applying ice during the first twenty-four hours after the injury will help stop the pain. If blood and fluid have accumulated under the nail (subungual hematoma), a hole can be drilled in the toenail, and the pressure and fluid will be released. The nail plate may be permanently damaged or deformed, however.

How Are Fungal Infections Caused?

Fungal toenail infections, or mycotic nails, can occur after years of microtrauma to the toe, as always, from shoes that don't fit right. When the nail matrix is infected, little can be done to correct it. Usually, your best bet is to have the nail surgically removed. Antifungal drugs can also be applied to the nail, and can be combined with periodic professional cleaning of the nail. A physician can do this. However, the nail never looks the same if the matrix has been affected by the fungus. Antifungal drugs may have side effects.

How Do Calluses Cause Foot Pain in Older People?

Calluses are the second most common condition (after nail problems) I see in older persons. Usually, they strike the areas under the tips of the toes, particularly the big toe and the little toe, sometimes on the side of the big toe, and the outer and inner borders of the heel. Painful fissures caused by the dry, thickened callus may also appear on the heels.

As you know, most calluses form around a bony abnormality in a mechanically unsound foot. A callus is nothing more than a buildup of hard, thickened skin that develops due to abnormal friction and pressures on the foot. Even gaining 10 pounds can increase callus formation.

How Are Calluses Treated?

The most conservative approach is to remove the hard skin by shaving down the callus tissue every four to six weeks. Then, removing excess pressure on the foot by using orthotic shoe inserts will change the abnormal forces on your foot. Often a measure as simple as wearing rubber-soled shoes can alleviate some of the callus symptoms.

What about Home Remedies?

When age has robbed your skin of some of its elasticity and moisture, it is important to try to restore this lost moisture. Before going to bed, soak your feet in lukewarm, sudsy water for approximately fifteen minutes. Then towel-dry them and rub in any type of moisturizing or hand cream. Apply the cream all over your foot, concentrating on the callused areas. Then cover your foot in plastic wrap, and put on a sock. In the morning, remove the sock and plastic wrap, and thoroughly wash your foot. Then use a pumice stone or a callus file (available in most drug stores for less than $2), applying a sawing motion to remove some callus. Make sure you only use this stone on thickened skin. (Another caution: If you have impaired circulation, diabetes, or nerve problems, avoid this treatment, for the combination of slow healing and too-vigorous scrubbing can lead to infection.)

What Will Help My Feet as I Grow Older?

Exercise—every conceivable kind: walking up and down stairs, cleaning, bending, all are important for aging feet. The most beneficial is walking at least thirty minutes a day.

Here are a few guidelines:

- Don't go barefoot if you have any neurological problem. The neurological system is not as intact as it was at age 25; thus, a cut that you may not even feel is susceptible to infection.
- Wear the correct type of shoes while walking (see "How to Choose the Right Shoes," page 176). Use jogging shoes for your daily walk. Remember that the cushioning effect of the shoe is very important: you should never feel as if you are "walking on pebbles."
- Watch out for obstructions in your path.
- Walk only where there is good lighting. As we grow older, our eyesight just isn't as good as it once was, and it's much easier to trip and fall.

Most foot problems must be treated conservatively, such as with shoe modifications, heel padding, and custom-molded shoes. Orthotics of latex, leather, plastic, or foam rubber can be very effective.

However, when conservative treatment fails to relieve foot pain, surgery can be considered. If you are in excellent health, age shouldn't be a barrier to effective treatment with surgery. When possible, local anesthetics should be used.

I have tried to include the most common foot problems older patients may face, although there are many more. Regular exercise will help prevent injuries and accidents, for weaker muscles often mean less resistance to injury. Remember, your painful feet can limit your ability to enjoy an active, independent life. If you take care of such problems, in the words of the poem, the best years *may* be those "yet to be."

More Exercises for Older Feet

Here are a few other types of exercise that may be helpful:

- Walking a minimum of fifteen minutes a day, progressing to one hour three times a week. Walking should be brisk.
- Skipping rope starting with five skips a day and working up to fifty.
- Aerobic exercises. Thirty minutes of aerobic exercises, at any level, can make you feel ten years younger.

Chapter 28
Let Your Feet Let You Feel Good

Have you ever had a day when your pains and troubles seemed to settle in your feet? All you wanted to do was go home and soak them. Next time, do more than soak them.

Here is what you need to know about foot massage, reflexology, pedicures, and the sex life of the foot.

Massage Your Feet for Their Well-being and Your Own!

Massage is, first and foremost, a great relaxer. It stimulates circulation while relaxing muscles, thereby giving instant relief to tired, sweaty, swollen, itching, or blistered feet. Massage can also offer temporary relief for foot cramps caused by ill-fitting shoes or overactivity. Cold, numb feet will quickly feel warm again after a brisk massage.

Massage is especially useful after surgery on the foot. I use it as a form of physical therapy on my postoperative patients, and it works wonders. Massage increases circulation to the injured area, and this increased blood supply helps speed recovery. It also relaxes muscles that have retracted excessively or been damaged. Massage also reduces the swelling that is present after any physical trauma to the foot such as an injury or operation. Swelling indicates an increase in the activity of the lymphatic system, and massage reduces the swelling by moving these lymph fluids back toward the heart. Removing the swelling takes pressure off the nerves of the foot as well and offers further relief.

Giving Yourself a Massage

It's easy to give yourself a foot massage. Start by warming your feet. There are several ways to heat feet, ranging from the ultraluxurious to the simple:

- For a truly lazy foot treatment you can buy a commercial device that not only bathes and warms your feet but massages them too. Automatic controls allow you to adjust the heat and the tiny massaging vibrator fingers to comfort.

- You can create your own foot whirlpool by sitting on the edge of the tub and allowing running water to soothe and stimulate your feet. Try starting with warm water, slowly increase the temperature and then decrease it again, using whatever extremes are necessary to make your feet feel tingly and fresh.

- If the bathtub whirlpool doesn't sound relaxing to you or seems to require too much effort, a good old-fashioned foot soak in lukewarm water with or without Epsom salts is also the perfect remedy for modern ills. You can even make it a luxury depending on what foot preparation you indulge in. Always give your feet at least fifteen minutes to soak in lukewarm water. This gives you a head start on your massage by dilating blood vessels in your foot, which in turn increases circulation and relaxes the muscles.

- Another way to give your feet a preliminary heat treatment is with a heating pad, but be careful, it can burn the skin on cold feet with poor circulation.

- I find that hot, moist towels offer the most effective massage preparation. Soak two or three towels in very hot water. Using first a dry towel wrapped around your foot to protect the skin against burns, alternate layers of hot wet towels and dry towels. Continue alternating through as many layers as necessary to hold the heat in. Then sit still for fifteen or twenty minutes, and let the heat do its job.

Beginning the Massage

Once your feet are feeling warm and relaxed, sit with one leg crossed over the other with the meaty sole of the foot facing you. Your thumbs are your massage tools. Use both of them in deep, circular motions, concentrating on very small areas at a time. Use various movements to discover what works best and slowly make your way from the tips of your toes to your heel. All movement, and the greatest pressure, should be *toward* the heart, to help move the "stagnated" circulation back to your heart, not away from it. Continue working in this direction from your toes to your ankle to your calf.

Try to find the areas that are knotted up. (You may already know—only too well!—where they are.) An area may be very sensitive, and you may even feel a tiny obstruction in it. This is due to adhesions: fibrous tissue deep in the ligaments or muscles. Some of my patients tell me that they feel small tumors underneath the skin, but these are not, in fact, tumors. They are just overworked muscles on the sole of the foot. Kneading the bottom of the foot will cause these bumps to diminish and eventually disappear.

After you've worked on stimulating the deep tissue and muscles of the sole of the foot, give some attention to the top of the foot. Reverse your hand position and use your thumbs—gently on the soft skin here—to stroke the top of the foot. Try opening the foot. With your fingers under the sole and the thumbs on top beside each other, gently squeeze the foot and draw the thumbs away from one another. This stretches the tendons that lie there.

Here are some other techniques to add to the basic massage:

- Pinch along the outside edges of the foot.
- Slap the sole lightly, with a relaxed wrist.
- Pound the sole lightly with a relaxed wrist and fist. Stroke the foot afterward to soothe it.
- Wring the foot, one hand above the other as if it were a sponge, by twisting it in opposite directions, slowly and firmly. Do this up and

down the foot from the ankle to the toes, using as much pressure as possible.
- Work the toes. Grasp each toe between the thumb and forefinger and give it a slow, gentle tug. Wiggle it from side to side. Think of the "This Little Pig Went to Market" game.

Finally, switch feet!

Experiment with what feels good on your own feet. Pamper yourself often with a warm footbath and a massage. You may also want to expand your foot massage into an overall body massage. You may even want to swap foot massages with a partner!

THE TWENTY-MINUTE PEDICURE

From start to finish, this simple routine shouldn't take more than twenty minutes. Yet your feet will feel wonderful for your minimal efforts.

1. Soak your feet in lukewarm water and vinegar for several minutes.
2. Dry them thoroughly, especially between your toes.
3. Cut your toenails straight across and don't clip into the corners. Keep the nails straight and simple. Nails should be squared off and trimmed without using an emery board. Don't cut them too short. Use a regular nail clipper. No scissors, please. Choose a clipper with a straight edge. Don't pick your toenails, and clean only the tips of the nails; avoid digging along the sides.
4. If you have a lot of callused tissue, soak your feet in camomile tea that has been thoroughly watered down. For calluses around the heels, or on the balls, apply a mixture of crushed aspirins—fifteen of them—mixed with a tablespoon of water and a tablespoon of lemon juice. (For more homemade foot fixers, see Chapter 31.) Make a paste of this mixture and apply it to all the hard skin on your feet. Put a warm towel over your feet and sit for ten minutes so the paste will have a chance to penetrate. When you remove the towel, try a pumice stone or soft brush on the calluses.
5. A little mineral oil, baby oil, vitamin E oil, or vitamin A and glycerine massaged into your feet will make them feel great.
6. Nail polish can come next if you like.

Reflexology: Taking Massage One Step Further

Reflexology is a theory and practice based on foot massage. It is purported not only to make the foot feel good but to improve the health of other parts of the body as well. According to this theory, such a long-distance effect is possible, because there are points on the foot which affect other organs and parts of the body. Working these reflex points, as they are called, keeps the whole body in a good state of health.

Reflexology was introduced to the United States in the early 1900s by a medical doctor, William H. Fitzgerald. Dr. Fitzgerald divided the body longitudinally into ten zones with each zone ending in one of the ten toes. With this organization he theorized that all organs lying in the same zone affected one another. For example, since the kidneys and eyes share zones, working the reflex points of one could help the other. Dr. Fitzgerald coined the term "zone therapy," and from this, reflexology was born.

Given the number of nerve endings in the foot leading back to the spine and other parts of the body, this theory may have some scientific support. As of now, however, there is no scientifically accepted explanation for the success of reflexology. While I am not an advocate of reflexology and don't understand how it could possibly work, it is worth mentioning here. Like acupuncture, acupressure, and hypnosis, it does seem to yield positive results in certain suggestible people.

How Reflexology Works

Reflexologists not only divide the foot into ten long zones incorporating all the parts of the body, but into shorter, horizontal zones as well. The short zones correspond to the trunk of the body. Imagine a person in the shape of two feet and you have a general idea of what a map of reflex points looks like (Figure 28-1).

To make it even more complicated, the foot is a three-dimensional map chock-full of reflex points, and one organ—the liver, for example—may lie across several different zones

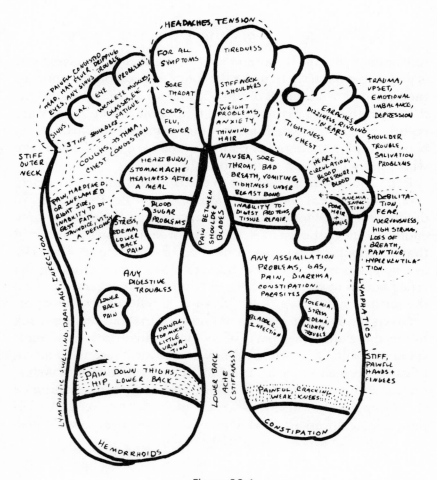

Figure 28-1
Reflexology chart of common ailments.

and have a number of corresponding points. The toes are especially crucial, as congestion or clogs there, at the tip of an energy zone, can disrupt everything else in the same zone.

A reflexologist begins by giving the feet a thorough going over. While this may look like massage, and even includes massage, the reflexologist is actually working particular points on the foot's surface. Using his or her thumb, the reflexologist moves in tiny steps trying to locate points that may be as small as

$^1/_{16}$ inch. Each pair of feet is different. The points that emerge as problems are then scratched (as if they were "itches") with tiny strokes of the thumbnail. The reflexologist searches for grainy deposits that may be impairing the flow of energy in the body and works them out, noticing at the same time what organ has been impaired. Sometimes a patient's reaction to pressure on a certain point will reveal where a potential problem lies.

A good reflexologist works with three goals in mind: (1) to improve transmission along the nerves and in the circulatory system, (2) to relieve tension, and (3) to balance the flow of energy in the body.

This last aim is most important, as reflexology is based upon an idea of maintaining a balanced distribution of what is sometimes described as a life-force, which must be free to circulate among all parts of the body. Working the reflex points helps keep the all-important end points in the toes and feet clear.

After giving the patient's feet a complete treatment, the reflexologist returns to the reflex points of any organs that are giving the patient problems and gives these points special attention. Without accepting the basic premises of reflexology, these treatments sound ridiculous. A sore throat, for instance, is treated by rotating and pulling the big toe. Anemia is treated by rubbing the inside edge of the foot. Stimulating the ball of the right foot keeps the liver ticking smoothly.

Where to Find (or Become) a Reflexologist

Going to a reflexologist for forty-five minutes twice a week isn't going to hurt you. It may not help you either. Reflexologists are not yet required to be licensed in the United States. They walk a very fine line between doctors and masseurs, and they know it. Most books on reflexology will not speak of healing the body because, legally, that claim can only be made by a doctor. Instead, reflexologists prefer just to work the reflex points of specific organs without drawing any conclusions about their effects. While they admit that their routines do improve general good health, they won't hazard a guess why.

Thanks to the interest in reflexology awakened in the seventies, it is fairly easy to find a reflexologist through a massage or holistic healing center. If you want to learn the art yourself, there is an International Institute of Reflexology in St. Petersburg, Florida. The institute is run by Dwight C. Byers, nephew of Eunice D. Ingham Stopfel, one of the early reflexology pioneers. The institute offers two-day seminars all over the world to teach reflexology. After completing the seminars, and practicing for one year on family and friends, students are permitted to take a test and become certified by the institute as reflexologists. Over 25,000 students have completed the course.

The Sex Life of the Foot

Don't laugh. Feet have long been considered a uniquely sexy part of the body. The Indian art of lovemaking includes toe kisses. Footprints in certain cultures served as love charms, and, if ever found, the footprint of the Egyptian goddess Isis was said to banish infertility. Feeling aroused to the tips of your toes is no exaggeration either. Alfred Kinsey, the noted sex researcher, has gone on record saying that after the most obvious signs of sexual arousal "the next most noticeable involve the feet and the toes. The toes of most individuals become curled or, contrariwise, spread when there is erotic arousal." Growing out of this natural interest in feet, foot fetishes abound and are said to outnumber other fetishes 3 to 1.

So how can your feet improve your sex life? That depends upon where and when you happened to be born. In China, for centuries the erotic appeal of small feet was so great that women's feet were bound. But did you know that this practice had a basis in historical accident? The club foot of Empress Ta-ki (1100 A.D.) inspired a decree that all women's feet should look like the foot of the empress. From then on, young girls, starting when they were five or six years old and continuing until they were adults, had their four small toes bent under the ball of each foot and bandaged tightly. This effectively shaped the foot's natural growth into the much-sought-after "lotus foot." While

Chinese men found the enforced delicate and teetering walks of the women exciting, the women themselves suffered intense pain. Foot-binding endured until the liberation of China in the twentieth century.

Neither small feet nor unsteadiness in walking as an ideal is restricted to the Chinese. A slender foot, able to fit into a glass slipper, distinguished Cinderella from her ugly stepsisters. For generations of children raised on this fairy tale, a small foot symbolizes feminity. We have Catherine de Medici (1519–1589) of France to thank for the introduction of high heels. Like the bound foot of the Chinese, high heels give women a mincing, provocative stride, and, once skirt lengths went up, helped create the illusion of longer and slimmer legs. The popularity of high heels has endured, and getting her first pair of heels marks a girl's important rite of passage into adulthood.

WHAT YOUR SHOES REVEAL ABOUT YOU

Do you wear loafers? Sneakers? Are your heels sensible or sensational? Does what you wear on your feet depend upon the state of your mind and mood?

Shoes say a lot about the person wearing them. After all, you consider more—much more—than mere comfort when selecting a pair of shoes. Shoes can signal playfulness, dependability, or even sexual availability. To some extent all clothes carry a hidden message, but shoes seem to have a special significance, especially for women. This may be a psychological phenomenon; Freud declared that shoes were symbols of the vagina. Certainly shoes have long been associated with fertility customs, marriage, and romance.

So how does all this relate to the kind of shoe you choose for yourself? Do your shoes unveil the real you? If you are a woman, find yourself in this list of "shoe personalities" and decide.

- The *Fastidious Woman* chooses neat, attractive footwear carefully matched to her clothing. She only buys shoes in her size—never yielding to the only-pair-left-in-blue-but-two-sizes-too-small temptation—and keeps them well-polished.

- The *Sensuous Woman* prefers open or deeply cut shoes to reveal the cleavage of her toes. She likes summer shoes and evening sandals best, with soles as thin and straps as narrow as possible.
- The *Sexual Woman* blatantly flaunts her feet in bright-colored patent leather or jeweled shoes. She often combines two kinds of materials—plastic with leather, say, or leather with satin. None of her shoes seem to be made with walking in mind.
- The *Working Woman* appears at the office. Knowing full well what connotations shoes carry, she avoids misunderstandings by wearing classic styles in neutral colors. Her shoes are elegant and understated.
- The *Withdrawn Woman* uses her shoes as an excuse to avoid facing the rest of the world. Her shoes are invariably inappropriate—mukluks in the summer, tennis shoes in the rain—and, if at all possible, she'd prefer to stay at home in slippers.
- The *Traditional Woman* favors the type of shoe she grew up with. No matter how styles change, she sticks with penny loafers or white sneakers or whatever. Anything out of line with her sense of style is considered cheap, tacky, or faddish.

Even men's shoes have significance. Heavy, thick-heeled boots are as much a statement of masculinity as sandals are of feminity. And, if you believe the advertisements, any of a number of competing brands of sports shoes can make a man stronger, faster, and more virile.

THE POLITICS OF SHOES

Given the silent statements our shoes make about us, it's no wonder that women's shoes have aroused comment. Why, asks the women's movement, are unsteady, unsturdy, and even dangerous shoes considered attractive? What makes high, thin heels, platform shoes, and flimsy sandals so popular? These shoes all seem to be missing the characteristics that make a shoe functional and comfortable. Think about it: "sensible shoes" for women are considered no fun.

One could argue that these sorts of shoes merely accentuate already existing female traits, adding an extra hip wiggle or extending the line of the leg. But others will point out that such shoes instill a sense of insecurity in women, and, by comparison, make men sturdier and more competent. And even if most women declare that they enjoy wearing high heels, it doesn't change the fact that as you can see in hard-core bondage magazines, spiked heels symbolize something not completely harmless.

Asking why women have submitted to various kinds of foot dis-comfort over the centuries—from foot-binding to platform shoes—goes straight to the heart of feminist concerns. Attitudes are starting to change. Although women still enjoy impractical shoes, they can also wear comfortable shoes without any adverse comment. If shoes are, in fact, an indication of who we are, then easily enough we can use them to make statements of who we'd like to be and how we would like the rest of the world to see us.

Chapter 29
Shoe Sense

Back in the Napoleonic era, soft, heelless slippers were in vogue among aristocratic French ladies. One day the Empress Josephine was said to have approached the royal shoemaker in distress. It seemed her brand new slipper had developed a hole in the bottom. The shoemaker carefully studied the slipper, then came to a startling conclusion. "I see what it is, Your Highness," he exclaimed, "you have *walked* in them!"

Fortunately, shoes today are designed to endure more than one wearing. Even so, many of us feel just as frustrated as the empress must have about the practicality of the trendy shoe styles we favor.

Shoes Across the Ages: From Greeks to Gucci

If you think back through time, you can see that shoes have nearly always had some kind of significance to society outside of their utilitarian purpose. In many cultures, a person's shoes have been a key to class or status in society. As far back as 1325 B.C. the Egyptians were adorning their sandals with elegant jewelry. In ancient Rome, only the aristocrats were privileged to wear sandals; slaves and servants went barefoot. In medieval Europe, the upper classes could be recognized by their long, pointy-toed shoes. These so-called poulaines or crackows originally evolved from a superstition that pointed shoes rendered witches powerless! As the custom caught on, the shoe points grew longer and longer—the longer yours were, the higher up you were on the social ladder. Aristocratic lords and ladies wore shoes with points as long as 12 inches that were so cumbersome they had to be pinned up to allow movement!

Political and economic conditions also have an effect on shoe styles. Consider the plain, peasant-like shoe worn by the French ladies after the revolution, in a time when anything smacking of blue blood could mean losing your head! Or notice the sturdy, simple shoes worn by the practical American Pilgrims as a result of their rugged lifestyle.

Shoes can tell us something quite literal about social mores and values. A ridiculous style of platform shoe worn by Italian women in the sixteenth century was a way, according to some sociologists, to keep women "on a pedestal." Walking in these 2-foot-high wonders called *chopines* was next to impossible, and it kept women frail and dependent. Eventually the shoes were banned, as the danger of a pregnant woman miscarrying became evident.

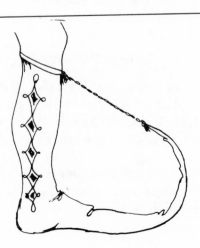

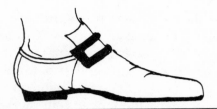

In prudish Victorian times, when flashing your ankle was considered scandalous, shoes weren't much to look at. What good was a beautiful shoe if no one could see it under your gown?

Thank goodness we don't go to these extremes today. But shoes still mirror what's going on around us now. Luckily for our feet, the sports craze has made athletic shoes more popular. Wearing these comfortable shoes while doing the shopping, or while commuting back and forth to your job is definitely "in"! (That trend is rumored to have started in New York City when the subway went on strike several years ago. Practical women who had to walk to work all the way from Brooklyn wore their tennis shoes, and never took them off.) On the other side of things, however, high-heeled, dress-for-success shoes are back with a vengeance. In the elegant eighties we're into designer shoes that show status and class—and if we don't choose wisely, our feet pay the price!

Getting Shoe-Wise

I have patients who come into my office with shopping bags full of expensive shoes, asking *why* they can't get shoes that don't kill their feet! Some despair of their "odd"-shaped feet that shoe salesmen have convinced them just don't fit into "normal" sizes.

Having your feet feel good *doesn't* mean you've got to wear clunky orthopedic shoes your whole life. I myself love to wear attractively styled high heels. What we could all use is a little shoe sense—knowing the basics on how to get a shoe that *fits* you! Certainly some shoe salesmen lack training in this area. So it's up to you to know what's right for your feet. Before you go on to read the next section take this little Shoe I.Q. Quiz. How many of these shoe myths have *you* fallen for?

MYTH: Shoes need to be "broken in" after you buy them.
MYTH: Orthopedic shoes can correct foot problems.
MYTH: Leather is always the best material for all parts of a shoe.
MYTH: The best heel for a shoe is no heel.

How did you do? A lot of us have suffered, literally, from such misinformation about shoes. I remember limping around miserably in brand new penny loafers when I was a child, trying to "break them in." Sure, it eventually worked—after my foot was all blistered and sore; but it wasn't necessary. Time and time again my patients ask me questions about shoe fit, and they walk out of my office a little more savvy. It may seem like a lot of fuss to learn about this, but your feet will thank you for it.

The Parts of the Shoe

Before we start, let's get our shoe vocabulary down. Let's look at a typical woman's shoe, the pump, to get a feel for the parts of a shoe.

Insole: The inner layer on which your foot rests.
Outsole: Also known simply as the sole, it's the shoe's bottom layer.
Upper: The part that is visible as the top of the shoe all around your foot. This is the part that largely determines the shoe's character.
Toebox: The reinforced area in the shoe's tip which shapes the shoe and protects the foot.
Heel: A solid projection down at the back of the shoe on which the shoe rests.
Shank: The part of the sole between the heel and the ball.
Quarter: The back portion of a shoe's upper.

The one element you don't see listed here that has a lot to do with a shoe's characteristics is the *last*. A last is a plastic or wooden model of a foot, over which shoe material is stretched

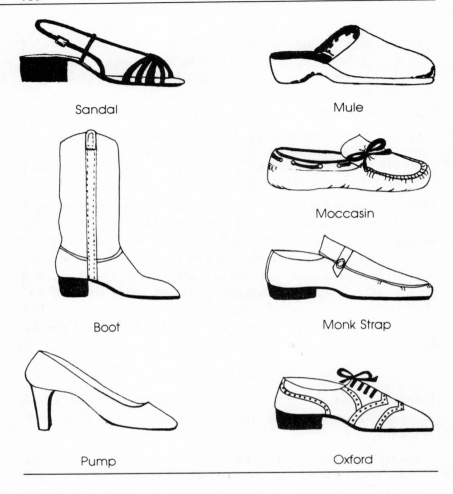

Sandal

Mule

Boot

Moccasin

Monk Strap

Pump

Oxford

to create the form. Each shoe designer has a special series of lasts with which to work. The process of stretching the leather over this form is called *lasting*.

Though it seems there is an incredible variety of shoes on the market, shoes today are really just variations on seven basic shoe types, some of which have been with us for centuries.

Mocassin: Hide or leather wrapped around the foot, with a very loose construction. It rivals the sandal for the oldest known shoe type.
Sandal: Basically just a sole, with no upper, strapped to the foot.
Mule: A backless slip-on shoe, like a clog or a slipper.

Boot: Any shoe that extends up over the ankle.

Monk: A slip-on shoe with a wide strap that is fastened, often by a buckle.

Oxford: A lace-up shoe that came from medieval England.

Pump: A lace-less shoe that fits snugly to the foot, thus requiring no straps.

Questions My Patients Ask

I'm Confused About Shoe Sizes—Mine Always Seem to Vary. How Do I Know When I've Got the Right Size?

If you've ever popped into a shoe store and picked out a pair of shoes just on the basis of stated size, you know how deceptive shoe sizes can be! Sizes vary from manufacturer to manufacturer, because each is working with a different set of lasts. It's a good idea to become familiar with a few favorite shoe lines, but try on the shoes you're going to buy. Even if the shoe salesman brings you an identical shoe in another color, try it on. Even individual shoes have slight variations. Also remember that your feet are different sizes depending on the time of day and the weather. It's best to try on shoes at the end of the day, when your feet are slightly larger as a result of swelling. They'll be larger in warmer weather, too.

What Can I Do If My Feet Aren't the Same Size? Is This Normal?

Just because shoe designers make shoes in pairs doesn't mean that our two feet are identical! Each of your feet is as individual as you are. So don't feel strange about it—take comfort from the fact that most peoples' feet aren't the same size. If one of your feet is larger than the other, resist the urge to cater to that smaller, more delicate looking foot. Though you may be able to squeeze that right foot into a size 6 at the shoe store, it'll start to hurt you later! Always buy for the *larger* foot, and ask the shoe salesman to give you a cushioned insert for the smaller one.

I Don't Have Any Problem with Sizes, but I Can Never Find a Shoe That's the Right Width. What Should I Do?

Many people forget to take width into account when sizing up a shoe. Shoe widths are labeled with letters; the narrowest is AA and the widest going up to D or EEE. Just like size, widths vary with the line of shoes. Knowing the general shape of your foot to begin with will help. This may sound obvious, but it's amazing how many people fail to consider the shape of their feet when they go shopping for a pair of shoes. Don't be a square peg in a round hole; the more you go against the natural shape of your foot in shoe selection, the more likely you are to end up with foot pain. So, for example, if you've got a prominent instep, avoid a shoe with a tongue that rubs against it. Instead, try an open-toed variety, or an unconstructed shoe that will leave it pressure free.

For those of you who despair of your wide feet, knowing different lines of shoes will save you hours of time and disappointment. Being aware that your feet are wide and that imported Italian shoes are usually narrow, you can eliminate them as possibilities. When you do find a line of shoes that fits you, stick with it! And keep praying that more manufacturers will wake up to the fact that we're not all petite AAs!

Are There Any Specific Shopping Tips on How to Tell If a Shoe Fits Properly?

The first rule of thumb for deciding if a shoe is for you is sheer common sense: does it feel good? Don't believe any salesperson who tells you the shoe will stretch, or that you have to break it in. The shoe should feel good now! Here are some things you should be sure to check:

- Make sure the ball of your foot rests on the widest part of the shoe.
- Your heel should fit snugly, and should not slosh around in the shoe.
- Toes shouldn't push or bulge against the top of the shoe—make sure you can wiggle them. The space between your *longest* toe (not necessarily your *big* toe) and the shoe tip should be at least ½ inch. If

your toes tend to develop corns, make sure you look for a high toe box.

- Don't just check the fit sitting down—walk around!
- If you do end up taking home shoes that you're not absolutely sure about, test them further at home. Wear them around the house with a pair of socks over them to keep them dirt-free. Then if there's a problem, you can still return them.

Do I Have to Give up High Heels to Be Comfortable?

Even if you have felt an aching sensation in the balls of your feet after running around town all day in high heels, you don't necessarily have to give up those shoes! My philosophy about heels could well be applied in other areas of living: "Moderation!" That means saving those 2-inch-high Ferragamos for a night on the town or an important business meeting.

First, figure out what moderate heel height is right for your everyday shoes. Most foot experts recommend a heel somewhere between ¾ and 1 inch. The proper height for you is the lowest you can wear with comfort. This doesn't mean the lowest heel possible, though. Heelless shoes can cause knee pain, particularly when you have shortened calf muscles. To find a good heel height for you, try touching your toes; if you can't reach them, you've got short calf muscles and should probably take a heel on the higher side. If you can touch your toes with ease, a flatter shoe is more appropriate for you.

The trick I use for making sure my feet don't suffer the effects of high heels is to change my shoes throughout the day. (I always keep a pair stashed in my office desk drawer.) I alternate a pair of lightweight, flexible leather shoes like loafers or topsiders with my high-fashion shoes. I put them on while I'm sitting at my desk working. If you alternate heel heights, you won't stress any muscle group unduly, and the muscles in your calf don't shorten and cause bad posture which can add to your foot pain.

Always keep a shoe's function in mind. It's fine to have several pairs of taller heels for fancy occasions, but also build a solid repertoire of basic office pumps, as well as comfortable shoes like loafers, oxfords, sandals, and sneakers to lounge around in. I think it's great that women are wearing sneakers around the city, when they're on the go, and saving their heels for the office or where their feet aren't unduly stressed.

What Are the Best Materials for a Shoe?

This depends on what you're going to be using your shoes for. The choice depends on weighing the following characteristics: breathability, flexibility, and durability. And certain materials are better for certain parts of the shoe, depending also on function.

Upper: Leather has traditionally been considered an ideal material for shoes, and as far as the upper is concerned, it may still be your best choice. Although man-made materials are now used in about 35 percent of all American shoe uppers, leather is superior. It looks better than synthetics like vinyl because it's so smooth and supple. These same qualities make it very comfortable. Leather conforms to the shape of your foot, stretching with use thoughout the day, and is a porous material that lets feet breathe. Leather, of course, is more expensive than other materials, but for looks and comfort, may be well worth the price. Don't forget that there are different grades of leather, too; some look better than others.

Vinyl and urethane are often used in the uppers of less expensive women's shoes. They're more durable than beautiful, and they lack breathability. It's probably best to stick with them for foul-weather boots. A material called porometric is a more sophisticated synthetic that breathes better and is good for an everyday shoe. The softer and more flexible your upper, the easier it is to wear the shoe.

Insole: Again, with an insole you have to decide what's most important for your foot. If you've got sweaty feet, you'll need the moisture absorption that leather provides. An average pair of adult feet gives off about ⅛ *pint of moisture* per day. The moist, dark environment of your shoe is a perfect breeding ground for bacteria and fungi, which can lead to skin infections. If an insole isn't porous, your shoe can harbor foot odors! But again, leather adds to the expense of the shoe. So if sweat isn't a problem for you, you may want to stick with a synthetic insole. A note of caution about cheap insole materials: the salt from your perspiration may begin to eat away at them, causing the insole to crack or curl.

Most manufacturers skimp on the cushioning of the insole necessary to protect your foot. The best solution is to put cushiony inserts into your shoe. The foam variety that you pick up at your local drug store is not as effective as Spenco insoles (nitrogen-impregnated foam) or so-called PPT ones (porometric foam). They're more shock absorbent, and last longer; you can even wash them.

Sole: Think about it: the sole is the only thing between your foot and that hard pavement. Jolts that are not absorbed by the sole go straight to your knees, hips, and lower back. Back when human beings ran around on the bare earth, they didn't need shoes to protect their feet. But we moderns experience about 1000 tons of impact through the ground daily! You need a sole that can absorb some of that force.

Rubber and crepe are excellent shock absorbers, though they tend to get gummy on hot days. Leather works, too, but leather soles are usually too thin—you feel every pebble beneath you, and these soles wear out fast. Polyurethane is a good alternative, and is the most widely used sole material. It's lightweight and flexible, and more durable than leather.

Heel: Since your heel absorbs 25 percent of your weight, it needs to be very sturdy. Just as important for shock absorbance and balance is the heel lift. Synthetics are often too slippery, and leather is too delicate. I recommend a rubber heel lift.

How Can I Tell a Quality Shoe?

Look for the following as a sign of a well-made shoe:

- A good shoe often has a rigid shank of steel, wood, or leather beneath the arch for support. Check to see if the midsole of the shoe is flexible; if so, it won't be very supportive.
- Look for the Goodyear welt method of shoe construction. Rather than having the sole and the upper directly sewn together, both are sewn to a rib or welt of material, often leather.
- Check the back and sides of the shoe for a counter, a piece of stiff material that adds heel support.
- Run your hand along the inside lining to find possible irritants—loose linings, wrinkles, lasting tacks, or any ridges between the sole and sides.
- Make sure the stitching is neat. No loose threads or missed stitches! Stress points should be double-stitched.

Is Shoe Upkeep Important?

Taking care of your shoes will not only keep them looking attractive longer, it will keep them working for your *feet* longer.

- Polished leather stays softer longer. Before I wear new leather shoes, I always spray them with a leatherguard.
- Don't wear the same pair of shoes every day. Give your shoes, and your feet, a breather from bacteria and offensive odors the shoe may harbor. If you have to wear your shoes two days in a row and your feet sweat, stuff them with newspaper to soak up the moisture. Cornstarch inside also keeps them dry.
- Use shoe and boot trees to retain the shape of your shoes.
- Don't neglect those heels! Run-down heels mean uneven walking patterns and poor posture, not to mention a ruined shoe. Never let an exposed heel drag against the hard pavement. Go to the shoemaker and have a tip put on.

Chapter 30
Weather Tamers

Your feet are incredibly sensitive to the conditions around you. As the weather changes from season to season, your choices of shoes and foot- and leg-related apparel should change, too. For the health of the feet, it's wise to know what toll the weather can take on you and how to respond.

Sun and heat can provide exhilarating freedom for your feet. Walking barefoot on the beach is a great way to exercise the *intrinsic* muscles of the foot (small muscles originating in the foot that control the toes). Sandals offer an attractive and comfortable alternative to the heavier shoes of colder months: they aerate the feet, which is especially advantageous for those who perspire heavily. Because sandals do not constrict the foot, problems such as blisters, bunions, and hammertoes tend to be alleviated with properly fitting sandals.

You should be careful of exposure to the sun—and certainly of overexposure—if you suffer from any kind of connective tissue disorder, diabetes, and certain superficial skin conditions which are prevalent on the lower extremities. In the heat, there is an expansion of lymphatic fluids and thus a greater tendency for swelling. For those with soft tissue injuries or ankle sprains, it may take longer for swelling to subside in the summer months. This is also true for people with postoperative swelling: with the increased heat, a return to normal size may take longer. The extent to which this happens varies according to one's own body chemistry.

If you're wearing a closed-up style of shoe in the summer, try to get something in a natural fiber. While they are durable and easy to clean, synthetic materials do not breathe like natural materials, and they may cause the feet to become overheated and uncomfortable. Also, synthetic materials do not give or stretch but always keep their original shape. Acrylics and polyester in socks and shoes should be avoided by people susceptible to athlete's foot. Of the natural materials, cotton and leather create the best environment for feet, while rubber and wool may induce sweating and retain moisture.

Cold, on the other hand, causes constriction of the blood vessels, which diminishes any kind of healing. Anyone who knows someone suffering from arthritis also knows that cooler weather tends to affect, sometimes acutely, the arthritic condition. Frostbite and chilblains occur when feet are allowed to become wet and cold so it's important, during the winter months, to keep feet warm and dry. Be alert to numbness. Keep your feet moving when you're outdoors. When you come in from the cold, give your feet a massage to restore circulation. Soak feet in tepid water or expose them at room temperature until they warm up.

Be sure feet are well-protected against cold and wetness outdoors by wearing water-resistant boots with thick soles. Boots should be roomy so they don't restrict blood circulation. Thermal cushions, or thick, fleecy insoles inside the boots, may be added for extra warmth, and perhaps two layers of loosely fitted socks.

Humidity is perhaps the most important climactic change to be aware of. When the barometer rises, any bursal sac or inflammatory condition that you have may become distended or exacerbated; the resultant pressure on the nerves can cause increased pain. Dampness also adversely affects most arthritic and painful chronic conditions.

Here are some of my thoughts on certain special kinds of foot- and leg wear:

Boots.   One has to be very careful to find precisely the right fit in boots, or the extra constriction may result in poor circulation. A lot of boots also impinge on certain deformities such as bunions and hammertoes, and may cause blisters and irritation.

Be aware of how high the boot comes up on your legs. This is very important. The calf is the thickest part of the lower leg and, as such, may be quite vulnerable to constriction. When constriction occurs, fluids in the lower leg tend to pool: it is difficult for the fluid to flow properly, and it may be restrained in its movement back toward the heart. Waterproof boots are made of nonporous material and are not designed to be worn all day.

Leg Warmers.   These help relax the muscles. By increasing the heat in the legs, leg warmers make it easier for the legs to be stretched and are appropriate for certain warm-up isometric exercises and for aerobic classes. They are particularly recommended if you suffer from muscle tightness.

Tights and Panty Hose.   I don't like the synthetic tights. I prefer the natural, durable fibers, those which don't constrict the blood flow or cause irritation to the skin. Pantyhose are fine but, here again, you have to be cautious about synthetics and how they constrict. I advise against stockings because of the garters, girdle belts, or girdles needed to hold them up—your blood flow can easily be impaired.

Socks.   I like cotton socks best, ones that do not constrict too much or those that go up to the knee. Find socks which were designed to fit your feet: the notion that "one-size-fits-all" in socks is ridiculous.

How to Keep Shoes Clean

It's not only your feet and your legs that take beatings in severe weather; your footwear does, too.

You can keep leather shoes clean by brushing them with a dry brush to remove dirt. Wipe with a damp cloth to remove dried-on dirt; then let the shoes dry away from any direct heat source. To remove scuffs, apply a paste wax of the same color as the shoes. Buff vigorously with a soft cloth (old socks are ideal); then brush to a high shine with a clean, dry shoe brush.

Patent leather shoes can be wiped clean with a slightly damp cloth. A very light application of petroleum jelly will keep your patent leather from drying or cracking.

For suede or pig suede, brush with a stiff brush to remove the surface dirt. An art gum eraser will remove everything but oil stains. Don't use paste wax on suede.

A water-repellent spray is useful in winter to keep shoes (and, hence, the feet) dry, and to retard salt deposit stains which have a tendency to occur in snowy weather.

Shoes for All Seasons, Please!

A lot of people complain that it's difficult to dress fashionably *and* sensibly, and I agree that the weather can present problems. You miss your stockings and heels when there's slush on the street or freezing temperatures in the air. But the comfort and the health of your feet must come first. If it's snowing, doesn't it make sense to wear a pair of warm, roomy boots? Sandals in summer, while great for some people, can be uncomfortable for others—be your own best judge. Sneakers are the ideal footwear for many athletic activities or when you're going to be doing a lot of walking, though whether you find sneakers the last word in fashion or not is a matter of personal taste.

My point is this: Dress appropriately. To feel comfortable is attractive in itself. If you merely go with the latest style, the pain may show on your face. And after all, how fashionable is it to walk with a limp?

Chapter 31
Foot Care Products

Miss America was once sighted touring the country with her lovely clothes, her beautiful hairdo, her crown . . . and her corn pads.

In the 1979 Grand Prix Master's tennis tournament, a painful foot blister forced Jimmy Connors to default, losing his chance to win the $100,000 first prize.

This list of the famous and glamorous with foot pain could easily go on. No matter how exalted the company you keep, you may still need a cure for your foot pain. A quick peek into any drug store's foot remedy department will show you just how much business the search for foot relief generates.

Last year alone, Americans spent more than $200 million for over-the-counter remedies for foot problems. Of this total, $47 million went for athlete's foot remedies, which I discussed in Chapter 12, and a whopping $86 million was spent on salves and pads. The sad thing is that most customers probably got only temporary, or inadequate, relief for all that pain.

Some products (like the antifungal sprays, ointments, and creams for athlete's foot, for example) are genuinely helpful. And those who seek only relief from shoe pressure will get it from the safe, simple pads and cushions they buy. But now the druggist is also stocking medicated pads, acidic liquids that "remove" foot problems like corns, calluses, and warts and more, and solutions that supposedly convince ingrown toenails to "grow out." While all of these products have some merit, most people don't know enough about what the product *really* does (and doesn't do) for them or what it could do *to* them if they used it incorrectly.

In this chapter, I'll take a look at some of these products, compare prices with value, and try to clear up some of the confusion. This list is not all inclusive; it's a sampling of what you might find if you decided to search the shelves for a remedy.

I'll also give you some suggestions for remedies you can make yourself. And, at the end of the chapter, I'll tell you what you can do to regularly keep your feet in tip-top shape.

I want to issue one important warning, however, before I list any products: If you suffer from diabetes or poor circulation, *always* consult a doctor about painful foot problems of *any* kind. Don't attempt to cure them yourself, even with products rated as "safe" for most people.

Diabetes affects small blood vessels throughout the body, and can result in decreased circulation and decreased ability for wounds to heal and resist infection. So even foot conditions that are minor problems for other people can present a great danger to people with diabetes and circulation problems. Any injury to the feet of such people can result in a very bad infection.

A final word: When you see the words "clinically proven to cure" on any product, what that means is not that that particular *brand* has passed standard tests (although it probably has, if it's a major company), but rather that its *ingredients* have been repeatedly tested and have won approval from the Food and Drug Administration (FDA) as safe and effective for the problem in question. In other words, if two different brands have different packaging promises but contain the same ingredients, they will be equally effective in helping your pain or growth.

Corns

Most medicated corn (and callus) products contain salicylic acid, an ingredient which an FDA expert advisory panel has rated as safe and effective. This medication, however, must be used very carefully: You must apply it only to the problem area, keeping it away from the surrounding healthy skin, on which it could cause burning and ulcers.

When you apply these products to a corn, it's a good idea to put a corn pad (doughnut-shaped) around the corn to protect the adjacent skin. The FDA panel also advises against using a salicylic acid product for more than five treatments and recommends that you see a doctor if the corn shows no sign of improvement after two weeks. When using any of these medicated products, it's best to apply them overnight, when foot perspiration is at a low, and about twice a week.

With these cautions in mind, here are some of the corn reliefs available to you:

Dr. Scholl's Liquid Corn/Callus Remover. This is packaged as a bottle of 12% salicylic acid, plus pads to go around the affected area. It is relatively inexpensive, safe, and effective, as long as you keep it away from normal skin and don't use too much.

Dr. Scholl's Corn Salve. This is a 15% salicylic acid cream marketed in small jars of approximately 4 fluid ounces, sold with pads. It is quite expensive. The same precautions apply.

Freezone Solution. Similar to the Scholl product, this is a 12% salicylic acid liquid, approximate size, ⅓ fluid ounces, and quite expensive.

Dr. Scholl's Corn Removers. These are pads with "disks" of medication, 20% salicylic acid, dispensed in packages containing twelve pads, and quite expensive. "Waterproof" pads cost about 10 cents more per package of twelve and have a higher (and potentially more dangerous) percentage of salicylic acid (40%).

Dr. Scholl's Corn Cushions. Relatively inexpensive, these come with and without wrap-around tabs. They do *not* contain medication and will not cure your corn; they only provide relief from friction against other toes and the shoes. They do what they purport to do, and do it quite well!

One warning, though: Don't wear corn cushions or pads for too long.

They can irritate the skin, and lengthy pressure around the corn can cause the exposed part of the center to rise even higher, possibly bumping into the top of the shoe. Also don't put a bandage around a corn; it won't relieve the pressure, and it will take up valuable room in shoes.

Dr. Scholl's Lamb's Wool (or any other brand). Lamb's wool is nonallergenic and good for sensitive skin. It is used for corns between the toes and its purpose, like the pads, is simply to relieve pressure on the affected area. The wool should be placed between the involved toes. A package, typically 3 × 4 inches in size (containing an abundant quantity of lamb's wool), can usually be found at a fairly low price.

Dr. Scholl's Corn File. This is a flat, plastic stick with a rough substance on the top half, and it works just like an emery board. If you use one of these, I recommend that a moisturizer be used first. However, "sanding down" one's corn with this kind of product rarely produces any satisfactory results; you're not going to make the corn go away, and you may hurt yourself!

Calluses

Many calluses are normal and need no treatment; after all, the function of a callus is to protect sensitive skin from pain. However, if you have calluses that are thick *and* painful, you should find a treatment for them. If you have a cracked callus, see a doctor, because the opening in the sore invites infections. If your calluses aren't painful but their appearance bothers you, you can also have them removed; however; I'd advise you to live with them.

As with corns, products that claim to be "callus removers" contain salicylic acid, and all the same important precautions must be taken in using this strong kind of medication.

Dr. Scholl's Pink Medicated Disks. These are relatively inexpensive, but are nevertheless quite strong in medication. The disks consist of 40% salicylic acid. To avoid blisters, and possibly ulcers, apply these disks very carefully to only the yellowish area of the callus.

Dr. Scholl's Liquid Corn/Callus Remover. See above under "Corns."

Dr. Scholl's Callus Reducer. This is a studded stainless steel file with a plastic handle and, like the corn reducer, it is used as an emery board to "file away" calluses. It is effective in making calluses smoother, but is generally more expensive than the pumice stone, which in my opinion does just as well. (Warning: individuals suffering from diabetes and poor circulation should not use this product, since any slight cut could result in a disabling infection.)

Dr. Scholl's Callus Cushions (or any other brand). One can usually obtain this product in one of two forms: either doughnut-shaped, for calluses on the tops of toes, or smaller solid pads, for calluses on the bottom of the foot. Both forms help to reduce friction on the callus but do not completely eliminate the callus. Doughnut-shaped cushions are generally available in packages of six; the pads are typically sold two to a package.

Dr. Scholl's Moleskin (or any other brand). Moleskin is made of sheep's wool. It is a nonallergenic substance which provides padding for calluses. Sold as a roll (usually 7 × 31 inches) at a moderate cost, moleskin is typically self-adhesive and can be cut to size for placement directly over the callus. This product serves only to reduce friction.

Dr. Scholl's Vi-Foam Cushions, Dr. Scholl's Ball-O-Foot Cushions, Dr. Scholl's Full Inner-soles ("foam cushion"). These products (and any other brand innersoles) are grouped togeher because they do essentially the same thing—not much at all! Such pads are designed to cushion the bottom of the foot from friction against the shoe; they only work well when they are not tightly compressed. Although they are inexpensive, most pads, especially those made of foam, compress almost immediately. Some innersoles are also available in rubber. Rubber innersoles take up less shoe space and last longer than their foam counterparts but in my opinion, they are quite useless, since by their very nature they are tightly compressed.

Your best bet, if you're going to use a standard-sized, store bought insole is a felt pad. The felt pad won't compress as quickly as foam pads under the weight of your body. However, no two feet are alike, and for this reason a foot specialist is advisable. The foot specialist can provide insoles which correspond to the actual shape (and needs) of a particular foot. It is best that the padding be applied to the shoe instead of to the foot, since feet sweat and most padding tends to stick to the foot.

Bunions

Bunions are serious business, and you can't make them disappear with simple home remedies. If you have a bunion, you should see a foot specialist; it's that simple. There are, however, two kinds of products on the market which can provide temporary relief from shoe-induced friction and alleviate some of the pain:

Dr. Scholl's Bunion Cushions (or any other brand). These cushions act as a barrier between the bunion and the shoe. They are relatively inexpensive.

Any kind of Molefoam. These pads of foam serve to protect bunions from friction. Unfortunately, they must be replaced frequently—every one or two days—since they become compressed (and therefore quite useless) in a fairly short period of time.

Ingrown Toenails

There is no such thing as a true ingrown toenail "remover" that is sold over the counter. Ingrown toenails are generally a chronic, recurring (and therefore permanent) problem, and are best treated by a foot specialist. There are, nevertheless, a variety of products available to the public that claim to provide instant relief:

Dr. Scholl's Ingrown Toenail Reliever. This product contains sodium sulfide, which softens the offending nail and the skin around it, and thereby relieves pain. This is its only use. It is sold as a liquid in jars containing ⅓ fluid ounces; it is quite expensive.

Outgro Solution. Contrary to its name, Outgro Solution does *not* cause an ingrown toenail to "grow out." If you have a chronic ingrown toenail, it is often the fault of the nail's curvature. This product, which consists of tannic acid, chlorobutanol, and isopropyl alcohol, merely softens the afflicted area. This softening of the nail relieves pain in the same manner as Dr. Scholl's Ingrown Toenail Reliever. However, Outgro Solution is usually somewhat more expensive.

An antibacterial cream, Bacitracin is truly helpful for ingrown toenails. While Bacitracin doesn't correct the problem, it does help to prevent infection and irritation which often accompany ingrown toenails. It is an inexpensive product which pharmacies sell without prescription.

Warts, Athlete's Foot, and Foot Odor Problems

Wart products should contain salicylic acid; athlete's foot remedies should contain either acetic acid or tolnaftate; and foot odor treatments should contain aluminum chloride hexahydrate. For details concerning individual products, please refer to Chapters 11 to 13.

Miscellaneous Foot Care Products

Dr. Scholl's Toe-Flex. This is an oval-shaped piece of hard rubber that is placed between the big toe and the other toes. It is intended to straighten crooked and overlapping toes. Unfortunately, products such as Dr. Scholl's Toe-Flex (which are relatively inexpensive) do no such thing; there is no effective home remedy to correct crooked and overlapping toes, which are biological deformities. This kind of product can be quite painful to wear. It can also result in greater friction between the toes and the shoe.

Dr. Scholl's Flexo-Foam Arch Support. This is one of the more expensive products in the Scholl line of foot products. It does not hold up for very long, nor does it provide permanent relief for pronated feet.

Dr. Scholl's Spring Arch Supports (or any other brand). Such supports are made of metal, are quite uncomfortable, and often prove to be too hard on the foot. I recommend that you avoid this type of product completely.

Dr. Scholl's Therma-Cushion Insulating Insoles. This type of product doesn't "warm" the foot as well as one might hope. Furthermore, it has the same "compression" disadvantages that are found in other insole products. A warmer pair of socks would probably provide greater comfort.

Effective Remedies You Can Make

Throughout this book, I've offered my own little "recipes" for the treatment of various foot ailments. The following additional home remedies are offered here for your consideration:

For Callused Feet Soak your feet in camomile tea that has been thoroughly diluted. It will stain your feet, but the stain can easily be removed with water. Camomile tea is generally found in grocery stores.

For Foot Cramps Run water in your bathtub at a cool temperature (about 60°F), and put your feet under the flow for a minute. Then change the temperature to lukewarm (about 103°F), and keep your feet under for three minutes. Now you're ready for a massage. After a good rubdown, splash on a little witch hazel or rubbing alcohol. Dry your feet, and use a moisturizing lotion (for choices and values, see "Foot Beauty" at the end of this chapter).

For Sweaty Feet   One good method for keeping feet that sweat in their shoes cool and dry is to treat the *shoes*—sprinkle them inside with talcum powder or cornstarch. To treat your feet, have first a very cold and then a very hot footbath. This procedure constricts the blood flow to your feet, reducing perspiration. Then fix yourself a third footbath of ice cubes and lemon juice. Finally, rub your feet with alcohol. In hot weather, when your feet perspire, this form of treatment should probably be repeated every day.

For Extrasweaty Feet   Try a soaking solution of kosher salt (larger crystals than ordinary table salt) and water (about ½ cup of salt per quart of water). Be sure to powder your shoes.

For Warts   Try making a paste of crushed vitamin A tablets and aspirin and applying it directly to the wart. Then add crushed vitamin E.

Here's another suggestion from William Dvorine, M. D.* Make a saturated salt solution by adding ordinary table salt to water, stirring vigorously, until added salt will no longer dissolve. Soak feet for thirty minutes every night for a few weeks.

If your wart-relief measures don't reduce pain, do see a doctor.

For Brittle Nails   Apply lanolin or petroleum jelly daily.

For Fungus on Your Feet, Especially between Toes   Start with a tablespoon of baking soda in lukewarm water. Rub that on

---

*A Dermatologist's Guide to Home Skin Treatment, Scribner Book Companies, New York, 1984, p. 114.

the site of your fungus or bacterial infection, and then rinse and dry thoroughly. Finish off the treatment by applying powder or cornstarch.

Foot Beauty

Now that we've reviewed all the ailments of the foot, let's turn to ways to make the foot as attractive as it can be troublesome.

The problem is that most Americans don't even care for their feet, let alone think of them as part of their beauty regimen. (In other countries, completely different attitudes prevail: In Sweden, for example, 95 percent of the population take regular footbaths as part of their daily grooming practice.) But healthy and young-looking feet can be a source of pride for anyone.

First of all, here are some general steps of preventive foot medicine that you can easily practice:

1. Change socks daily, and wash nylon stockings thoroughly.
2. Don't wear the same shoes two days in a row. On one pair's day off, use your normal spray deodorant on them to kill bacteria and give them a dusting of cornstarch.
3. If you have a choice, pick cotton socks over nylon. Cotton allows feet to breathe better.
4. In warmer weather, try to wear sandals occasionally, to expose your toes to air and to help reduce the amount of closed-in perspiring your feet do.
5. If you regularly run or walk a good deal, put petroleum jelly on the tops and bottoms of your toes. It will help cut down on friction and will make your toes less susceptible to blistering.

Then try taking these three beauty steps if you want your feet to step out in style:

1. Soak feet in a sodium bicarbonate solution—1 tablespoon in 1 quart of water—or soak them in ½ cup of vinegar mixed with 1 quart of water. Both of these mixtures will make your foot surface more acidic, thereby cutting down on the amount of odor it produces. Take this kind of footbath twice a week for about fifteen minutes each time.
2. Use a moisturizing cream (see below) every day after bathing and

thoroughly dry feet. In addition, two or three times a week cover the moisturized foot with a plastic wrap and wear a sock over it, which will provide pressure and heat to help the cream penetrate into your opened pores. This treatment will keep the skin of your feet from drying out and will soften it enough for you to gently rub calluses with a pumice stone (after removing the sock and wrap!). When rubbing calluses, try to remove only a thin layer of dead skin each time, and stop if the callus starts to hurt or becomes inflamed.

3. Treat your nails well, too. You can use the same softening agent you use on your hands; massage it in thoroughly to soften and strengthen nails (this is especially important as you get older, because toenails grow increasingly brittle). Then clip your toenails. Always clip nails straight across; square corners will help prevent ingrown toenails. Use a *good* nail clipper—a sturdy, high-quality stainless steel clipper can cost about $10, but it's worth the investment. Finally, manually push your moisturized toenail cuticles back. This entire nail treatment should be done weekly.

There are a number of products sold in drugstores that are designed for use during such a regimen. I've found that few of them do anything a pumice stone and any moisturizer won't do. If you go looking for these "special" foot products, however, you may find some of these:

Dr. Scholl's Foot Beauty Buffing Cream. This contains water, paraffin, stearic acid, and glycenyl stearate, the same things you'll find in almost any moisturizing product. I think it's equally as effective to use your favorite hand cream, for instance, Ponds. Some generic brands of cream, which contain the same ingredients as all the others, can cost very little.

Pretty Feet and Hands. This is the name of the brand, not the guarantee. It will work as well as any cream, because it contains the same ingredients, but it will cost more.

Dr. Scholl's Foot Balm. This is like most creams and is especially similar in contents to Noxzema.

Dr. Scholl's Contoured Foot Beauty File. This beauty stick is coated with a rough substance and is curved to follow the contours of the feet. Everybody's contours are different, though, and the rough stuff merely acts as a pumice stone. The only real advantage of this product is its convenient handle, which gives good leverage.

Dr. Scholl's Foot Beauty Stone, Pequa Lady's Pumice Stone, or any brand of pumice stone. They're all the same; only prices vary.

Dr. Scholl's Foot Beauty Dual-Action Swedish File. This has two surfaces, one for merely dry skin and the other for hard calluses, but again, it just acts as a pumice stone with a handle. Basically, with a stone, *you* control how you deal with different levels of dry skin, by how and how often you rub or "file."

Johnson's Foot Soap. This is a box containing four envelopes of a powder made up of borax (for cleaning and soothing—boric acid smoothes skin), iodine (for working against bacteria), and bran (probably for texture). This doesn't do much any other formula of footbath won't do.

Dr. Scholl's Soap 'n Soak Instant Foot Bath. This contains sodium bicarbonate and soap, and you can really make it yourself, since you can buy sodium bicarbonate in any grocery or drug store. What this alkaline substance does is increase the acidity of your skin, helping your feet cut down on odor and resist certain organisms that might otherwise cause sweating.

My advice is simply to get yourself a good nail clipper, a pumice stone, and a moisturizer you like. The latter is especially important. Because of their location, the feet are the last area of the body to get your circulating blood supply, and therefore the skin is likely to become dry faster there than on other parts of the body. Almost everybody's feet have some dry skin.

Creams and lotions are equally effective as moisturizers for feet. General active ingredients include vegetable oils, mineral oils, lanolin, "wool fat" (the oil products of sheep, which are very smoothing and soothing), and collagen. (Warning: Some people are allergic to certain moisturizer ingredients, so before adopting any product, test it on a small patch of skin.)

All creams and lotions, since they are made of basically the same ingredients, work equally well; your preference should depend only on what packaging, scent, and feel you like. Another factor, of course, is what price you want to pay, since costs-per-ounce can vary greatly from one cream or lotion to another. The following is hardly an exhaustive list—just a sampling of some of the better-known brands of moisturizer you may already use or be tempted to buy:

Creams

Ponds Skin Cream. This contains mineral oil, petrolatum, glycerin, and stearic acid, and it's reasonably priced.

Nivea Cream. Same ingredients.

Eucerin Cream. Same ingredients, plus wool wax alcohol. Slightly more expensive.

Noxzema Cream. An all-time favorite that's a great buy. This contains camphor, phenol, eucalyptus oil, clove oil, and menthol, in addition to other ingredients.

Generic (your store's) brand. As inexpensive as Noxzema is, most large drugstores also sell their own, non-name-brand version that contains the same basic ingredients for an even lower price.

Almay Cream. Contains mineral oil, propylene glycol, and other ingredients that are in most creams. This is one of the more expensive of the popular products.

Lotions

Lotions contain the same combinations of ingredients as their cream counterparts. Only texture, convenience, and price differ. Here are some examples:

Vaseline Intensive Care Lotion. Inexpensive.

Nivea Lotion. Also inexpensive.

Jergens Lotion. Yet another good buy.

Almay Lotion. The price is steeper than others.

Lubriderm. A medium buy, but, I think, one of the better lotions available. Effective and nongreasy.

Now here are five of my personal favorites, the moisturizers I think do the most for feet:

Aquacare. Cream or lotion. This is a particularly effective product that contains a special substance called urea that attracts and holds moisture in the skin. This also contains petroleum, glycerin, lanolin, and mineral oils—the usual ingredients. It's expensive but worth the money.

Carmol. The same kind of urea product as Aquacare, although it absorbs a little better, and costs a little less. Like Aquacare, the cream is 20 percent urea, and the lotion 10 percent.

Hydrisinol. This is made with specially treated sulfonated and hydrogenated castor oil and with hydrogenated vegetable oil (which is the same thing as Crisco). It's a great treatment for dry skin. Hydrisinol is one of the more expensive products I'm recommending, but this, too, is worth the money.

Selectracream. Contains salt, mineral oil, and other ingredients common to most of these products.

Petroleum jelly. This, finally, is the best moisturizing product of all, in my opinion. It's also one of the cheapest. You can buy Vaseline or a generic brand for less money per ounce.

One final "do-it-yourself" product tip: It's not as pleasant to use as most of the above, but Crisco (yes, what's in your kitchen) is just as good a moisturizer as any cream or lotion on the market!

No matter what products you use, for purposes from pain to prettiness, what's most important is that you *pay attention to your feet.* If that means consulting a podiatrist for a severe problem, do so. If it means engaging in home treatment with a store-bought or homemade product, make sure you know what it is you're using and what you're doing. Once you start being nice to your feet, you'll be astonished by how much more cooperative they'll be with you.

Chapter 32
How to Find Someone Special for Your Feet

When to Use the Podiatrist and When the Orthopedist

A podiatrist is a specialist in the treatment of diseases, deformities, and injuries of the foot, whereas the orthopedist is a doctor who treats the bones and joints of the entire body.

With the running boom came a vast increase in foot ailments, and, in response to this, in the practice of podiatry. Many foot problems are now treated by the podiatrist.

In most countries, podiatrists are called *chiropodists* (those who care for the feet *and* hands). In the mid-1900s, chiropodists in this country began calling themselves podiatrists, to reflect their emphasis on the foot.

Originally, podiatrists were known as little more than "corn cutters." Their training was minimal. Today, however, things have changed drastically. A podiatrist-to-be must attend one of the country's seven podiatric colleges. Three to four years of undergraduate college are required for admission, and training at a college of podiatric medicine takes four years—the same as at medical school. Graduates receive a D.P.M.—Doctor of

Podiatric Medicine—degree, and usually enter a one- or two-year residency program for specialized training at an approved hospital, or a preceptorship. After successfully passing state and national examinations, the podiatrist is licensed by the State Board of Podiatry Examiners. The podiatrist can practice in any state after passing its licensing examination.

There are under 10,000 podiatrists in the United States, and the country's seven podiatric colleges graduate a total of approximately 700 new podiatrists a year.

Surgery has become the focus of podiatry's growing appeal—specifically, ambulatory versus hospital surgery. With ambulatory surgery, the patient can have virtually painless treatment in a podiatrist's office on a Friday, and be back at work—nearly pain free—by Monday.

The biggest barrier to widespread acceptance of ambulatory procedures, I think, is that people just don't believe surgery can be so simple. Bunions, bone dislocations, over- and underlapping toes, hammertoes, corns, nerve tumors, and a variety of toenail difficulties can be treated in a podiatrist's office. At the start of the procedure, novocaine is used, with a compressed air gun, into the area where it is needed. The patient feels a sensation similar to a mosquito bite. Then, a fast-acting local anesthetic is administered with a hypodermic.

A tiny incision, less than ½ inch, is made in the skin. A rotary file, similar to a dentist's drill, is placed under tissue and capsule directly on the site of the deformity. Then, using digital perception and a very fine instrument, the podiatrist explores the deformity and corrects it. Tendons and ligaments are generally undisturbed.

The whole procedure is similar to that used by a plastic surgeon performing a rhinoplasty (nose repair). Some instruments are the same in both procedures; there is no major incision, no general anesthesia, and a minimal scar. The smaller the incision, the greater the skill required of the surgeon. Most patients say the sensation experienced during minimal incision surgery (MIS) is similar to that felt during dental work. One knows the work is being done, but feels no pain. Afterwards, most patients do not even require aspirin for postoperative discomfort.

Normal wound healing generally occurs within a week. Usually it takes two months for the bone to heal completely. Swelling may not disappear for several months, varying with each patient.

By avoiding hospitalization and general anesthesia, chances of infection and other complications are greatly reduced. The patient saves hundreds, or even thousands, of dollars in hospital bills. Since MIS is so simple and painless, and relatively inexpensive, why do people continue to hobble around on aching feet? Because MIS, like so many other medical advances, will take time to catch on.

MIS is not a new technique. It became prominent in the late 1950s when Dr. Edwin Prober began teaching it to the podiatry profession. A renaissance in podiatry came about.

Ambulatory foot surgery is still controversial. Not unlike the debate which has raged for over a decade over "lumpectomy" versus radical mastectomy for the treatment of breast cancer, there have been violent discussions. Many orthopedists insist that foot surgery is their domain, and many hospital-based podiatrists flatly refuse to do in-office foot surgery. But good news has a way of spreading. People who have experienced ambulatory surgery tell their friends. Because it works.

I don't believe that there should be antagonism between the podiatrists and the orthopedists. Podiatrists see many more foot patients than orthopedists do; only a portion of an orthopedist's practice concerns foot care. Furthermore, podiatrists often work with orthopedists and will, on occasion, refer a patient to them. Orthopedists also receive referrals in the case of bone, muscle, or MMS (joint) problems that are symptomatic of generalized disease or traceable to other parts of the skeletal structure.

What about the New Sports Medicine Podiatrists?

There are also sports medicine podiatrists who examine and treat the various disorders common to athletes. Through biochemical evaluation, review of medical history, and clinical examination, the specialist can diagnose each foot type and all of the various disorders that are caused by the thousand natural shocks an athlete's feet are heirs to. The podiatrist may recommend a different pair of running shoes, exercises and stretching, orthotic devices, or, in some cases, corrective procedures to create a more efficient running style. You can learn more about sports specialists in your area by contacting the American Academy of Podiatric Sports Medicine, 2192 Martin, #100, Irving, California 92715.

How to Select a Podiatrist

How do you select a podiatrist? As with any other kind of doctor, recommendations—from a patient satisfied with the doctor's work, a hospital, another doctor, or even from reading material—are best. Sometimes, however, this process can prove more confusing and time-consuming than illuminating, especially when four or five doctors are on your list and you have the definitive lowdown on each. It is possible to overload yourself with opinions.

Always ask the podiatrist as many questions as possible—or, rather, as many as it takes you to feel comfortable with him or her. Have you established some sort of rapport with the doctor? What hospital affiliations does the doctor have? How many years of experience has the doctor had in treating the very problem for which you need help?

Only when your questions are answered to your complete satisfaction should you trust your feet to the doctor.

TRADENAMES

Below is a list of tradenames used in this book, together with the firms in whose names the tradenames have been registered.

Betadine, *The Purdue Frederick Co.*; Polysporin, Neosporin, Empirin with codeine, *Burroughs Wellcome Co.*; Bacitracin, *Pfipharmecs Division*; Whitfield's Ointment, *Eli Lilly*; Indocin, *Merck Sharp & Dohme*; Compound W, *Whitehall Labs, Inc.*; Buf-Puf, *3M Co. Personal Care Products*; Duofilm, *Stiefel Laboratories*; Gelfoam, Lotrimin, Tinactin, Celestone, *Schering Corp.*; Halotex, *Westwood Pharmaceuticals, Inc.*; Desenex Products, *Pharmacraft Consumer Products*; Johnson's Deodorant Foot Powder, Johnson's Odor-Eaters, Johnson's Foot Soap, *Combe, Inc.*; Quinsana Deodorant Foot Powder, *Mennen, Inc.*; Basis, Eucerin, Nivea Cream, *Beiersdorf*; Lubriderm, *Warner Lambert*; Meditar, *Ray Drug*; Hydrisinol, *Pedinol Pharmacal, Inc.*; Carmol HC, *Syntex Laboratories, Inc.*; Aquacare/HP, *Herbert Laboratories, Inc.*; Tylenol, *McNeil Consumer Products Co.*; Coumadin, *Endo Laboratories, Inc.*; Dexatrim, *Thompson Medical Company, Inc.*; Unna Boot, *Miles Pharmaceutical*; Butazolidin, *Geigy Pharmaceuticals*; Lysol, *Sterling Drug Co.*; Spenco Insoles, *Spenco, Inc.*; Dr. Scholl's Deodorant Refresher, Dr. Scholl's Deodorant Spray, Dr. Scholl's Liquid Corn/Callus Remover, Dr. Scholl's Corn Salve, Dr. Scholl's Corn Remedies, Dr. Scholl's Corn Cushions, Dr. Scholl's Lamb's Wool, Dr. Scholl's Corn File, Dr. Scholl's Pink Medicated Disks, Dr. Scholl's Callus Remover, Dr. Scholl's Callus Cushions, Dr. Scholl's Moleskin, Dr. Scholl's "Vi-Foam," Dr. Scholl's "Ball-O-Foot," Dr. Scholl's Full Insoles, Dr. Scholl's Bunion Cushions, Dr. Scholl's Ingrown Toenail Remover, Dr. Scholl's Toe-Flex, Dr. Scholl's Flexo-Foam Arch Support, Dr. Scholl's Spring Arch Supports, Dr. Scholl's Therma-Cushion Insulating Insoles, Dr. Scholl's Foot Beauty Buffing Cream, Dr. Scholl's Foot Balm, Dr. Scholl's Contoured Beauty File, Dr. Scholl's Foot Beauty Stone, Dr. Scholl's Foot Beauty Dual-Action Swedish File, Dr. Scholl's Soap 'n Soak Instant Foot Bath, *Scholl, Inc.*; Freezone Solution, Outgro Solution, Pretty Hands and Feet, *Whitehall (Ayerst Pharmaceuticals)*; Requa Lady's Pumice Stone, *Requa, Inc.*; Almay Lotion, Almay Cream, *Almay International*; Vaseline Intensive Care Lotion, *Chesebrough Ponds*; Jergen's Lotion, *Andrew Jergens Co.*; Selectracream, *Syosset Labs*; Crisco, *Proctor & Gamble.*

Index

About the Author

Suzanne Marin Levine, D.P.M., Dip: ABAFS, is one of the pioneers and leading practitioners in the technique of ambulatory, in-office surgery. Dr. Levine holds a Master in Physical Therapy degree and a Doctor of Podiatric Medicine degree from Columbia University and The New York College of Podiatric Medicine, respectively. Her postgraduate education was gained at New York University School of Medicine, Mount Sinai Hospital, and Astoria General. She is a member of The Academy of Ambulatory Foot Surgeons, Diplomate Board of Podiatry Examiners, Diplomate of The American Board of Foot Surgeons (Ambulatory Division), and The American Analgesia Society. Dr. Levine has written articles for numerous publications, has been a guest lecturer at the Pennsylvania Podiatry Association Conference, hosted a program called "On Your Feet" on New York City radio station WVNJ, and has appeared on T.V. She is also on the adjunct clinical faculty of the New York College of Podiatric Medicine. Dr. Levine is currently in private practice in New York City.